a story of
healing body
and spirit

MINDFULNESS
AS MEDICINE

SISTER DANG NGHIEM

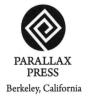

PARALLAX
PRESS
Berkeley, California

Parallax Press
P.O. Box 7355
Berkeley, California 94707
parallax.org

Parallax Press is the publishing division of Unified Buddhist Church
© 2015 Unified Buddhist Church
Printed in The United States of America
Cover and text design by Jess Morphew
Author Photo © Ron Forster
Illustrations and Photos © Sister Dang Nghiem except where otherwise noted in captions

Library of Congress Cataloging-in-Publication Data

Dang Nghiem, Sister, 1968-
 Mindfulness as medicine : a story of healing body and spirit / Sister Dang Nghiem.
     pages cm
  ISBN 978-1-937006-945 (paperback)
1. Dang Nghiem, Sister. 2. Meditation-Therapeutic use. 3. Healing--Religious aspects--Buddhism.
4. Suffering--Religious aspects--Buddhism. 5. Lyme disease--Patients--Religious life. 6. Buddhist
nuns-Vietnam--Biography. 7. Buddhist nuns--United States--Biography. I. Title.
 BQ950.A53A3 2015
 294.3657092--dc23
 [B]
                                        2015002143

2 3 4 5 / 19 18 17 16 15

In dedication to our Beloved Teacher
and his faithful transmission
of the Dharma through his life and practice.

In gratitude to Dr. Horowitz, Dr. Quang,
Gene Kira, Sister The Nghiem, Sister Truc Nghiem,
monastic and lay brothers and sisters.

To Sunee, the joyful manifestation
of my Mother, and my brother Sonny.

Each moment you live deeply is a love story.

CONTENTS

PREFACE   11

CHAPTER ONE   25   INTERBEING

CHAPTER TWO   79   FRIENDSHIP

CHAPTER THREE   115   JOY

CHAPTER FOUR   167   TRUST AND CONFIDENCE

CHAPTER FIVE   197   REVERENCE AND RESPECT

CHAPTER SIX   227   HEALING

CHAPTER SEVEN   303   ONENESS

ACKNOWLEDGMENTS   339

PREFACE

For seven years I lived in Deer Park Monastery in California, where we have many types of grand oak trees. Some oak trees have curved trunks and stretched out branches like graceful dancers. Some oak trees stand tall and upright with wide branches.

Wherever there are oak trees, there are also rocks and boulders. Over the years, an oak would grow over the rock and into the rock, and the rock would become a part of the oak and vice versa. If you ever see an oak tree that has fallen over, you will see that its deep roots are woven to rocks and gigantic boulders from underneath the surface of the earth. Rock and oak, they are two, but they have become one. They support each other. The rock offers the stability and the minerals to the oak, and the oak stands tall but deeply rooted in the earth and in the rock. This relationship between the oak and the rock is powerfully moving to me, and I believe that in true love we should be this to each other, that we should grow into each other over time. There is no longer the separation between you and me even though the oak has its own character and the rock has its own character. They live together in deep harmony and support. The oak can be oak because of the rock, and the rock can be rock because of the oak.

As spiritual beings together on a joyful path, we also learn to grow in our love, our transformation, and our healing in the spirit of the oak and the rock. Your happiness is my happiness, and your suffering is my suffering. Taking care of me is taking care of you, and taking care of you is taking care of me.

Few books talk about love for oneself. All of us want to love and to be loved, but we often direct this energy outward, focusing our love on a person or an object outside of ourselves. When we direct love outward in this way, we neglect the love that goes inward. Love becomes an idea of "self" vis-a-vis "other." It manifests a behavior of grasping, holding onto something to make it yours, in order to assure your chance of survival or to reinforce your sense of self.

What I have been going through in my life teaches me that love first and foremost must be turned inwardly. It must first be directed toward oneself.

As a young woman growing up, I always felt that if I had a successful career, if I became "somebody," and if I found my soul mate, then my life would be complete; all the losses and abuse I had experienced in my childhood would be compensated for.

I attained all of that. I went to medical school, had a successful career, and was young and beautiful with many people to pursue and many people pursuing me. I was also in romantic relationships. I had a partner who loved me absolutely—and yet I was always ready to turn my back on him every time the suffering of the past arose. I would befriend and cling to my suffering instead of cherishing the conditions of happiness available to me. I would look for love from the outside and I was never satisfied. Even if the Buddha came and loved me, I might still walk away because I didn't know how to love myself.

Often we think of a soul mate as a person outside of us who knows us well. In Vietnamese, the word "soul mate" is *tri ky*. *Tri* means, "to know, to remember, to master." *Ky* means "oneself." So a soul mate is one who knows, remembers, and masters oneself. As the word "tri ky" implies, it's important to remember that the true love—the soul mate we're always seeking—is already always present inside of us. If we know, remember, and master ourselves, we discover who we are, what the meaning of life is, and what we should be doing here on this planet Earth.

How can we learn this true love, to "know, remember, and master" ourselves? We can only master something if we know what it is and practice it often. In Chinese, the character "mindfulness" literally means "now mind" and it also means "to remember." Mindfulness has become a buzzword and a fashion nowadays. However, mindfulness in its true essence is an inherent human capacity. Daily mindfulness practice and cultivation strengthen this capacity to anchor the mind in the present moment, so that it can remember, know, and take appropriate care of the body, feelings, thoughts, and perceptions.

The Buddha used the image of the moon to describe the gentle, discreet, but ever-embracing quality of mindfulness. When the moon rises in the sky, it rises so quietly that it's unnoticeable. Most of us are not aware that the moon is rising. Even when the moon is already up there in the middle of the sky, most of us are still unaware of it. Yet when the moon is still at the horizon, it already starts to spread its soft gentle light and brighten the surroundings. As it ascends higher, the moon's light spreads farther and farther to the bamboo groves, to the forest, and to every small corner. Every part of life is being shined upon by the moon and is reflecting the moonlight.

This gentle, discreet, but ever-embracing quality of moonlight can be seen in mindfulness. Mindfulness is something soft, quiet, gentle, and discreet, but nevertheless it has the capacity to embrace all aspects of our life. It imbues every pore of our skin and every part of our being. When we're aware of our breathing, our steps, or a drop of dew that is hanging from the tip of a leaf, that awareness is gentle and soft like the moonlight. Yet it's ever penetrating and it brings a certain quality of brightness and lightness to us. We feel connected to that dewdrop, to that leaf, to that in-breath and out-breath, and to every aspect of our life. Quietly and slowly, we feel connected to life itself.

Thus, mindfulness practice has enabled me to cultivate and offer love to myself so that I will have something to offer to others, and so that when others offer love to me, I don't reject it out of fear or grasp it out of loneliness. Love shouldn't be from neediness or grasping, but from mutuality, understanding, acceptance, and trust that we offer to one another. Only then can love be true; only then can one have something meaningful, substantial, and real to offer to oneself and to others.

We're fortunate that the Buddha gave us four concrete teachings about the components of true love, which he referred to as the Four Immeasurable Minds of love, and which my Teacher, Zen Master Thich Nhat Hanh, also refers to as "the elements of true love." These are four capacities and qualities that are innate in each of us. Through our mindfulness practice, we can cultivate and fully realize them.

The first of the Buddha's Four Immeasurable Minds of love is *maitri*, friendship. This comes from the Sanskrit word, *mitra*, which literally means "friend." Every time my Teacher, affectionately known as "Thay" (which means "teacher"), talks about the Buddha's Four Immeasurable minds of love, he expresses a desire to retranslate their names. For example, the first element, maitri, has been translated as loving kindness, even though the root word, mitra, means friend. I would like to explore this element of true love and attempt to translate it as friendship or kinship.

The second element of true love is *karuna*, which means to help alleviate and remove suffering, either in oneself or in another person. Karuna has been translated as "compassion." I would like to explore this element of true love and translate it as "the capacity to heal" or as "healing." To heal is to become or to make something healthy or well again. Thus, healing can be seen as a process of transforming and removing suffering, so that well-being can be present in ourselves, in our relationship with ourselves, and with others.

The third element of true love is *mudita*, usually translated as "joy." Mudita may be the joy that we cultivate in ourselves or the joy that we offer to another person. When we're gratified by the joy that another person is experiencing, this is known as "altruistic joy," to feel happy for another person's advantageous conditions or achievements.

The fourth element of true love, *upeksha*, has been variously translated as "letting go," "equanimity," "nondiscrimination," or "inclusiveness." Because some people may associate the terms "equanimity" and "nondiscrimination" with equal rights, gender and racial issues, I would like to use the word "interbeing." In fact, interbeing encompasses equanimity, nondiscrimination, inclusiveness, and letting go.

During the Winter Retreat of 2011–12, Thay added two more elements to the Buddha's Four Immeasurable Minds of love. One is "trust and confidence." Among the several Sanskrit words for trust and confidence, I have chosen the word *vishvas*, which includes not only the meanings of trust and confidence but also the consequences that those elements bring: breathing freely, freedom from fear, confidence, reliance, comfort, encouragement, and inspiration.

The other element of true love that Thay has added is "reverence." I have chosen the Sanskrit term *nyas* for reverence or respect because its root word, *asyati* or *asati*, means "to put down upon the earth, turn or direct toward, deposit with, entrust or commit to, to place at the head, receive with reverence, call to mind, reflect, and ponder." Reverence is a capacity to recognize and to be in awe of what is.

In this book, I would like to share stories from my own life and practice and how I have applied these six elements of true love so that I may be a soul mate to myself and others. I also would like to approach them in a different order, starting with 1. upeksha, interbeing; 2. maitri, friendship and kinship; 3. mudita, joy; 4. vishvas, trust and confidence; 5. nyas, reverence and respect; and finally, 6. karuna, healing.

I choose to begin with upeksha because I feel that it's important to start with Right View; in the teaching of the Eightfold Noble Path, the Buddha also started with Right View. Once we begin with the Right View of interbeing in upeksha, all other elements of true love will be seen through this lens. Suffering is caused by ignorance, which is manifested as wrong views and wrong thinking. With Right View, healing and the other elements of true love manifest naturally.

In Vietnam, when two people cherish and love each other dearly, they may say to each other, "May we lose our teeth together." This statement reflects a deep desire to grow old together, when our hair and teeth are no longer intact and we're no longer physically attractive as we were in our youth. It also implies that each of us needs to learn to take good care of our own teeth, and the rest of our physical body, as well as mental and spiritual health, so that we don't desert the other person prematurely. It also means that we would do anything to help the other person to take care of his or her suffering and happiness and to cultivate wellness and endurance so that we can travel the long distance side-by-side.

Cultivating the Six Elements of True Love in ourselves is the most concrete practice that enables us to fulfill a lifelong commitment first to ourselves, which in turn enables us to understand, love, and live in harmony with our beloved and all others as well.

From my Teacher I have learned that every moment lived deeply is a love story. I wish to share with you some of these humble and nourishing moments. Through them, you will also have a window into the lives of our Plum Village monastic and lay practitioners. I hope you enjoy them, dear ones.

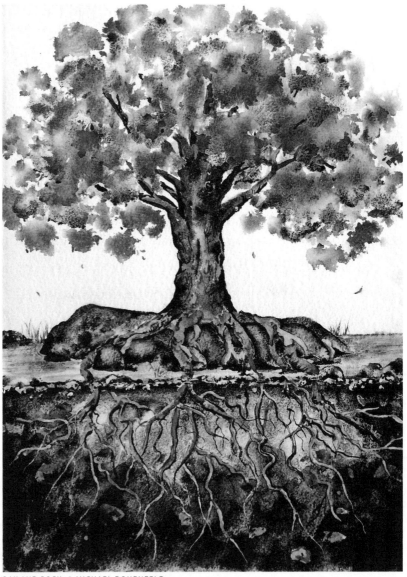

OAK AND ROCK, © MICHAEL DONENFELD

The Prajnaparamita Heart Sutra dates back from the beginning of the Christian Era. The heart of its teaching is that nothing can exist as a separate entity, but that all phenomena are products of dependent arising. This is in that. That is in this. This is because that is. This is not because that is not. This is indeed the Right View of interbeing. Unfortunately, the language used in the Heart Sutra and its previous translations have often caused the misunderstanding that emptiness means nothing really exists.

In August 2014, Thay was leading a retreat at the European Institute of Applied Buddhism (EIAB) in Waldbrol, Germany. In the midst of the retreat and his declining physical health, Thay's mind was crystal clear and powerful, and he finished retranslating the Prajnaparamita Heart Sutra as "The Insight That Brings Us to The Other Shore." This New Heart Sutra is Thay's invaluable gift to future generations.

THE INSIGHT THAT BRINGS
US TO THE OTHER SHORE

Avalokiteshvara
while practicing deeply with
the Insight That Brings Us to the Other Shore,
suddenly discovered that
all of the five Skandhas are equally empty,
and with this realization
he overcame all Ill-being.

"Listen Sariputra,
this Body itself is Emptiness
and Emptiness itself is this Body.
This Body is not other than Emptiness
and Emptiness is not other than this Body.
The same is true of Feelings,
Perceptions, Mental Formations,
and Consciousness.

"Listen Sariputra,
all phenomena bear the mark of Emptiness;
their true nature is the nature of
no Birth no Death,
no Being no Non-being,
no Defilement no Purity,
no Increasing no Decreasing.

"That is why in Emptiness,
Body, Feelings, Perceptions,
Mental Formations, and Consciousness
are not separate self entities.

"The Eighteen Realms of Phenomena,
which are the six Sense Organs,
the six Sense Objects,
and the six Consciousnesses,
are also not separate self entities.

"The Twelve Links of Interdependent Arising
and their Extinction
are also not separate self entities.
Ill-being, the Causes of Ill-being,
the End of Ill-being, the Path,
insight, and attainment
are also not separate self entities.
Whoever can see this
no longer needs anything to attain.

"Bodhisattvas who practice
the Insight That Brings Us to the Other Shore
see no more obstacles in their mind,
and because there
are no more obstacles in their mind,
they can overcome all fear,
destroy all wrong perceptions,
and realize Perfect Nirvana.

"All Buddhas in the past, present and future
by practicing
the Insight That Brings Us to the Other Shore
are all capable of attaining
Authentic and Perfect Enlightenment.

"Therefore Sariputra,
it should be known that
the Insight That Brings Us to the Other Shore

is a Great Mantra,
the most illuminating mantra,
the highest mantra,
a mantra beyond compare,
the True Wisdom that has the power
to put an end to all kinds of suffering.

Therefore, let us proclaim
a mantra to praise
the Insight That Brings Us to the Other Shore.

Gate, Gate, Paragate, Parasamgate, Bodhi Svaha!
Gate, Gate, Paragate, Parasamgate, Bodhi Svaha!
Gate, Gate, Paragate, Parasamgate, Bodhi Svaha!"

Chapter One

INTERBEING

One year on my birthday, a dear friend sent me some "Yin Yang beans." The bean has the usual oblong shape, but then it has a wavy line running down right in the middle, dividing it into two halves. One half is entirely white, but with a black dot; and the other half is entirely black, but with white dot. My friend ordered these beans online. They were called Yin Yang beans, but he named them "inter-beans." Perhaps the word "interbeing" sounds theoretical or mystical. These "inter-beans" say clearly: In this, there is that. In the white there is the black, and in the black there is the white. This is in that, and that is in this. It is what interbeing means. It's a concentration, a topic of constant meditation. As nuns, we wear the brown robe or the brown jacket, but if we think, "I am different from you. I am more special than you," then in that moment, we are not inter-beans, we are just beans!

For the first four years that I was a nun, I lived in the Plum Village Monastery in France, the place my root teacher, Thich Nhat Hanh, calls home. However, for many years now I've lived in Plum Village monasteries in the United States. Each day I practice walking and breathing mindfully, and finding the teacher in myself.

When I last saw Thich Nhat Hanh, he was on a visit to the United States and he was lying in a hammock, as he tends to do. I knelt down near him and gently pushed his hammock back and forth with my right hand. His skin was smooth and radiant, his eyes bright and serene.

After listening to him talk for a while, I asked him for a favor, to write down for me in his calligraphy: "True love begins with your body."

He asked, "Are you sure?" I looked into his eyes and replied, "Yes. That's what I have been practicing since I got sick."

I was able to look directly into Thay's sometimes-stern face, because I have learned to look directly into my own mind, recognizing and accepting its deviations, follies, and mischief. Thay's gaze softened and he said, "People often make a division between body and mind, but there is no separation between them."

My teacher, Thay, as his students call him, has taught me to love and to be loved in a way that it is true, beautiful, wholesome, and long-lasting. I have been doing my best to look into my passions and attachments in order to understand their roots and transform them gradually.

MY FIRST LOVE

My brother Sonny was the first person I learned to love in my life. Our mother was working in the market all the time. When we woke up in the morning, she was already gone. I would help him to brush his teeth. Then I would walk to the open market, which was only fifteen minutes away from our home, to buy some beef and lettuce. I would cut the beef into cubes, cook it lightly, and mix it with the lettuce. It was the easiest dish to make that I had learned from going to a French restaurant with my mother. That was our daily meal together.

Then my brother and I would bathe together before we walked to school. Our home had a floor made of cement and the drain was right there in the floor. The cement floor was very smooth. We had a big water jug right at the faucet for the water to run into. I poured water over the floor and then sprinkled powdered soap on it. My brother and I, both naked, would glide back and forth on this slippery floor. It was a small area, but we had great happiness playing this game almost every day. Then I would scrub the dirt off of his body, dress him, and walk him to school.

We slept together in the same bed with our mother. When our mother disappeared, my brother and I continued to sleep in the same bed. My brother would wet the bed every night. In our sleep, we would roll in the bed and then inevitably my head or face would end up on his wet spot of urine. In the morning my face would smell like urine, my hair would smell like urine, and my clothes would smell like urine. Every day I had to wash his clothes and my clothes. Irritation built up, and sometimes I couldn't bear it anymore.

This happened for years, and one day I got so fed up after having to wash our bedding I went out on the balcony to hang it up to dry, and as I did so I was screaming, "You wet the bed every night, on my head, on my face, and every day I have to do laundry and clean for you. God, please look down and pity me!" My brother's face turned crimson because he was already ten or eleven years old, and he had already begun to feel attracted to some girls in the village.

Many years later, when I came home from the monastery to visit him, we would have a heart-to-heart talk about our childhood. Throughout my college and medical school years, we did this every time I came to his place and stayed with him for a week or two. Our mother passed away when he was only eight, so I often told stories about our mother and about him so that he wouldn't forget her or his childhood. We would look at old photographs together. By this time, I was already a nun, and as we were talking, somehow that memory of me screaming on the balcony was brought up. He said, "Sister, when you were screaming like that I was very hurt, and until this day it still makes me sad." I looked at my brother and tears just streamed down. I told him, "I'm sorry, honey. I'm so sorry. Back then I was in a lot of pain and suffering too. I was also a child while I was trying to take care of you so I didn't know any better. Please forgive me, okay?"

It seems to be a trivial thing, but we'd carried it in our hearts, and it had continued to pain us. In that moment, as adults talking, laughing, and crying over it, we understood each other more and we also made peace with each other. It had never occurred to me to ask him why he didn't get up to go to the restroom, so I asked him then. He said he was afraid of ghosts; also it was so dark and a long way to walk downstairs to go to the restroom, so he just lay there and peed in bed. He was awake most of the time he did this. I told him if I had known that, I could have placed a pot next to our bed for him!

It is healing when we do Beginning Anew with ourselves and with each other. In the practice of Beginning Anew, we first acknowledge the positive elements in ourselves, then in the other person and in our relationship with him or her. We acknowledge our unskillful actions, the things that we've said or done to ourself or to the other person. Then we share what the other person may have done that caused us pain or confusion. In this process, we acknowledge our own pain. We see each other's pain. Your pain is my pain, and my pain is your pain. I learn to take care of my pain so that I can be happier. If I do everything I can to help you be happy, it also makes me happier. As a nun, I can't offer my brother money and material comforts anymore, but I know that when he thinks of me he feels at peace. He knows that I'm taking good care of myself and he doesn't have to worry about me. When he calls me on the phone, he knows I will listen to him wholeheartedly.

The unconditional love that I have given my brother over the years helps him to be the young man that he is. My brother still struggles to take care of himself, but deep in his heart he knows he is always loved by his sister. To be loved unconditionally by one person in your life is a great fortune. It helps you to move through the difficulty, loneliness, and despair in your life. There were times when my brother was a teenager that he held a gun against his temple and wanted to shoot himself because he saw no way out. Then he would think of me. He later recounted to me, "I would think about you, elder sister, and I would think that if I died, you would be all alone in this world and I didn't have the heart to do that to you. So I put the gun down." He did that for me many times. I, too, saved my own life because I, also, would think of my brother. That is the love that we can give one another. We think of each other's happiness more than our own happiness. We think of each other's suffering more than our own suffering. We try our best to take care of ourselves because we know that means the well-being of the other person.

DWELLING IN MY BROTHER'S COMFORT ZONE

While I was living in Deer Park Monastery in southern California, my brother used to drive from Arizona to San Marcos, California, to visit his girlfriend, who is now his wife and the mother of Sunee, my beloved niece. San Marcos was only twenty minutes away from the monastery. Once, when my brother called to let me know that he was stopping by to see me, I was so happy and I asked him if he had just arrived in California. He replied that he had been at his girlfriend's house for three days, and he added, "I can only stop by to see you for an hour." I asked him where he was going in such a hurry, and he told me that he had to take his girlfriend and her nieces and nephews to see a movie.

I was deeply hurt and saddened by my brother's action. Then a question suddenly arose in my mind, "How can I expect my brother to give me more than what he has?" Perhaps seeing me reminds him of our painful childhood, of his unfulfilled goals, or of my unconventional choice to be a nun instead of a doctor. If one hour is what he is able to give me, then let's rejoice in that one hour. If I were to expect him to give me more, he would be sad because he's not able to offer that to me, and I would be unhappy with what is. Then, both of us would be losing out.

Meditation is amazing. You may be in a situation year after year to which you always have the same reaction. But suddenly, in one moment you see something new, or you see the situation in a totally different way, and that breaks you free. The day-to-day practice of stopping and looking deeply culminates suddenly in this kind of groundbreaking, mind-liberating moment.

My realization may not have been that earthshaking, but it set me free. When my brother showed up, I asked him if he wanted me to go see the movie with him and the children. He was completely befuddled. He said, "I thought you couldn't go out of the monastery."

I told him I could ask permission from my elder sisters. He was really surprised and happy. From then on, whenever I could, I would go with him to his girlfriend's house. There were about ten children along with their parents gathering together at the house, and it was too noisy for me. My brother, on the other hand, was more at home in that environment than he was at the quiet monastery. Out of love for him, I learned to step out of my own comfort zone and accept what my brother could offer me. It set him free and he could be himself. It made me happy to see my brother happy. I played with the children and actually had a lot of fun with them.

SEPARATE COSMOS

There is a Vietnamese poem addressing the inevitable alienation one experiences in a romantic relationship:

> Even though we believe in one life and in one dream,
> You are still you, and I am still me.
> How can we cross over the one-thousand-mile wall?
> Both cosmos are full of mysteries.

When we have a child, at the beginning of our relationship with that child we may feel that our child and we are one. When the child is in the womb, mother and child are one. Then the child is born, the umbilical cord is cut, and the mother continues to care for the child. The life of the child depends on the mother and the father, so we continue to feel that oneness.

As the child grows up, he or she runs farther and farther away, and we experience a separation. This can be painful. In "the empty nest syndrome," parents whose children have gone to college feel that their home is empty because there are no longer children in the house. This separation feels as though something inside us is being severed. It can be excruciatingly lonely and painful.

When two people fall in love with each other, in the beginning they believe that they are one and will always share one life together. Unfortunately, in time, most of us discover that we're a different cosmos from the other person. Each cosmos is full of mysteries and these two cosmos may never meet one another.

This is why in many relationships we become more distant and grow further apart from each other. The pain, struggles, and difficulties build up higher and higher. There are days that we don't even want to look at each other or speak to each other. It's just too painful to talk about what has been going on.

But when we look in the light of interbeing, we see that each one of us truly does contain the entire cosmos, because we carry the experiences of our blood ancestors and spiritual ancestors as well as the experiences of animals, plants, and minerals.

All these experiences are inside us. In addition, during our lifetime, the way we think, speak, and behave also shapes and molds the person we are. If we see that each of us carries the whole cosmos within, then we realize that our personal cosmos isn't entirely separate or different from the others, and that all of them inter-are with each other. We may see them differently, experience them differently, interpret them differently, but they are all human experiences.

We isolate ourselves when we say, "I suffer, and nobody understands my suffering!" or, "My pain is greater than your pain!" As a result, we suffer alone. We push each other away, only to get lost in our own suffering. But if we look deeply, we will see that everyone suffers as a result of this wrong view.

If we could look at each other and realize that your suffering is my suffering, and my suffering is your suffering, and that we experience suffering and happiness more or less the same way physiologically and psychologically, then we would be more patient, more tolerant, and more embracing toward ourselves and each other. We would be more realistic in our relationship from the beginning. We could learn to share more openly and honestly so that we wouldn't be so easily fooled by our perceptions and expectations, and later on we wouldn't get so disillusioned with each other.

We know quite well that we are complicated. If we can keep in mind that we are a whole cosmos, that the other person is also a whole cosmos, then we can be more patient and loving, always making the effort to learn and understand each other. We'd be more cautious and take things more slowly. We would be more mindful, humble, and open with each other from the very beginning.

"I AM A FOOL"

At the end of our conversations, my belated partner John used to say, "What do I know? I know nothing; I'm a fool!" Then he would laugh joyfully. Actually, it was a joyful thing for us to say to each other when we were in good spirits and communicating on a deep level. I was the more serious one in our relationship. John didn't mind being "a fool," and it helped release the tension and made us laugh together.

I taught this to Sister Noble Truth—also known as Sister Noble "Tooth" because of the way she mispronounces her name when trying to say it in English. Apparently, she took my lesson to heart. Lay friends visiting the monastery would talk to her for a while and then wait for her response. Sister Noble Truth would say, "What do I know? I know nothing; I'm a fool!"

Lay friends were so surprised to hear this that they exclaimed, "No, Sister, you are not a fool!" Most of us certainly don't want to call ourselves fools. We want to appear smart, sophisticated, and knowledgeable. None of us wants to admit to ourselves that we are a fool, let alone claim to be one in front of others. It's frightening for people to hear somebody call herself a fool, so they react immediately by saying; "No, Sister, you're not a fool!" But she would insist joyfully, "Yes, yes. I am a fool."

One day Sister Noble Truth said this to a layman, but she mispronounced it, and it became "I know nothing; I'm a poo." The man stared at her in confusion. Later on in our room, Sister told me about that incident. I laughed so hard. Then I told her that there are different meanings of "poo." When you say, "I'm a Pooh, like Pooh Bear (she has a Pooh Bear in her possession), that's okay; it can be joyful. But if by accident you say I'm a poo, like in poo poo, it also means poop! So you really have to be careful." We laughed and she learned to correctly pronounce the words "fool," and "poo."

Another time during an orientation for a group of lay friends, Sister Noble Truth was invited to share. She said, "No, I just want to be here; I don't want to share anything." When we pushed her to say something, Sister Noble Truth said, "I know nothing; I'm a fool." Everybody was aghast. Sister Bamboo had to explain to the retreatants that our young sister had learned this phrase from me, and that this means a fool in the Shakespearean sense. This kind of fool is able to make fun of those who want to be sophisticated, the know-it-all aristocrats. Only the fool is able to make fun of them with impunity.

I think we should take on this role of the fool in our relationship. We have the saying, "I am a fool in love," but maybe we don't see it in quite the same light. One time John said to me, "I'm so in love with you. I'm so happy. I feel like my feet are walking on air." I replied, "No, I'd rather that you have your feet on the ground."

There was some wisdom in that statement, even though it turned out that I was the one who didn't know how to keep my feet anchored on the ground. When we're so in love that our heads are in the air and our feet are also in the air, then we can't see the situation clearly as it is. We may not take responsibility for our actions with mindfulness. We may not know what true love is. What we call love may just be infatuation. It may only be romance, passion, and pleasure.

Perhaps we can practice being fools, so we don't jump into the situation with our feet in the air, but we approach the relationship with more humor and spaciousness. We definitely should learn to make fun of ourselves. When we have strong feelings, even such feelings as love or attachment, we should ask ourselves, "You think so?" It's great when we're able to poke fun at ourselves.

This is not to doubt ourselves, or to belittle our feelings or perceptions. It's to give ourselves the space to question, to experiment, and to reexamine what is there. This helps us take the time and space we need to get to know ourselves and each other.

APPOINTMENT WITH SOUL MATE

As monks and nuns or lay practitioners, we do sitting meditation each day. In sitting meditation, we close down the five senses. The eyes are closed and don't take in or consume images. The ears don't take in sounds, like news, music, or conversation. The nose doesn't take in smells, like food or perfume. The mouth doesn't take in food or engage in conversation. Our body is still, stable, and upright, and we don't take in touch or have bodily contact with others.

Thus, we have only the mind to look at. Even with the mind, we quiet and calm it down by anchoring it to the awareness of the breath and of the body. When the mind is calm and still, it is able to look at itself.

In sitting meditation, we are actually making an appointment with ourselves. We learn to be our own soul mate, to be fully there and listen to ourself deeply. We are practicing the first mantra, "Darling, I am here for you," which means I am here for myself. I am here for the inner child in me, whether that child is three, five, or eight years old, a teenager, or a young adult who has experienced traumas, sadness, and joy.

In meditation, we use loving speech with ourselves, "Come back. Come back to the breath. Come back to the body. I am here for you, my love."

We ask ourselves with all humility and curiosity, "Tell me of your pain. Tell me why am I feeling so confused when this incident happens, when this situation arises? Tell me why it hurts so much to be with that person? Why does it hurt so much to be away from her?" Our speech is full of humility and love, and it's filled with a desire to understand ourselves.

Then, we listen.

Then, we gently ask another question for deeper understanding.

Then, we listen. We listen in order to make the connection with that child within. We listen in order to recognize that we are like this because our past experiences were like that. We are, because our inner child is. This is how we can learn to be our own soul mate. Deep listening and loving speech can be applied not only in sitting meditation but also in daily life.

We can also practice deep listening and loving speech while we're walking quietly, being fully aware of our steps and our breath. When the mind is aware of the steps, the breath, and the body, it is quiet, attentive, and spacious. If a thought or a feeling arises, the mind is able to perceive it and hear it. That is deep listening. We hear what arises in the moment, and we are fully there for it in that moment. We hear what is said and also what is not said. There is no preconceived notion or judgment. That is compassionate listening.

There are times when we hear somebody telling us something again and again, a hundred times, but because we think we know this already, we've heard it already, we finish the sentence for the person, or we readily draw a conclusion and the brain immediately closes down and doesn't process any more information, thus shutting out that person who is there with us. Our body is physically there, but our mind is already focused on another object, or it's planning, or daydreaming.

The other person feels this and knows that he or she is speaking to a wall. Sometimes the person may ask, "Are you there? Are you listening to me?" We reply, "Yeah yeah yeah, I hear you," but we've already shut that person out.

In the spaciousness and quiet of our mind, we may belatedly truly hear a familiar sentence for the very first time. We finally understand the message and ask, "Is this what you mean?" After all this time, five years or twenty years, we suddenly understand what our mother, father, or partner has been trying to tell us, and they may exclaim in exasperation, "That's what I've been trying to tell you all this time!"

We suddenly see how this message is connected to everything else. We discover this aspect of the person for the first time, and this is a moment of deep communion in our relationship, with ourselves, and with each other.

We need to practice loving speech and deep listening with ourselves first of all. The inner child in us, the deepest part of us, has been trying to tell us for so many years certain things about ourselves, but we just don't hear it. It's like being in a crowded and noisy market. Neither can we hear a voice calling us nor can we hear the sound of a pin dropping.

But when the market closes down and the cacophony ceases, if there's a child crying, we will hear it. In the same way, we need to cultivate this quietude in ourselves throughout the day, so that when the cries from deep down inside us rise up, we will hear them. We will recognize ourselves for the first time. We will understand why we are the way we are, why we behave certain ways. Only when we can do this for ourselves will we be able to do it for other people. Only then can we discover each other anew every day and in every moment.

Guided Meditation Exercise

The following guided meditation exercise can be used to befriend and heal the inner child in you, in your father, and in your mother. In this guided meditation, when you visualize yourself as a child, the child you come in touch with may be a child of any age—three, five, eight years old or a teenager. Accept this image of your inner child as he or she is. You can use this meditation frequently, and you may find you're in touch with different ages of your inner child in different sitting sessions. This is wonderful, too, because it allows you to acknowledge, embrace, and heal yourself at different stages in your life.

Instructions for Guided Meditation

In guided meditation, one line is recited for the in-breath and another line is recited for the out-breath. These two lines are followed by key words, which are a shortened version. The key words may help you focus your mind so that you can continue to follow your breathing as you practice looking deeply. Each guided phrase may last two minutes or however long it may take you to feel in touch and at ease with that part of the meditation. In the book *The Blooming of a Lotus* by Thich Nhat Hanh, there are several guided meditation exercises that you can use daily. Once you're familiar enough with this practice, then you can guide your own meditation.

Meditation is a bird with two wings—one is stopping and the other deep looking. In sitting meditation, we always start with stopping. We stop the mind from ceaseless thinking and aimless wandering by bringing the mind back, first to the breathing, and then to the body. Once the mind is anchored stably in the breath and body in the here and now, we can proceed to the second wing of meditation with a specific topic for contemplation.

Guided Meditation Topic: Embracing the Child Within

PART ONE: practice stopping by being aware of the breath

1. Breathing in, I am aware that I am breathing in.

   Breathing out, I am aware that I am breathing out.

   In-breath

   Out-breath

2. Breathing in, I am aware of the characteristics of my in-breath
   (short or long, shallow or deep, light or heavy, comfortable or
   uncomfortable, etc.).

   Breathing out, I am aware of the characteristics of my out-breath.

   Characteristics of in-breath

   And out-breath

3. Breathing in, I follow my in-breath from the beginning to the end.

   Breathing out, I follow my out-breath from the beginning to the end.

   Following the in-breath

   And the out-breath

PART TWO: practice stopping by being aware of the body

4. Breathing in, I am aware that I have a body.

   Breathing out, I smile to my body.

   Aware of body

   Smiling to body

5. Breathing in, I scan through my body from head to toe.

   Breathing out, I smile and send gratitude to each part of my body.

   Scanning body

   Sending gratitude to body

6. Breathing in, I am aware of the pain and tension in certain parts of my body.

   Breathing out, I smile and release tension from each part of my body.

   Aware of tension and pain

   Releasing

PART THREE: practice looking deeply

7. Breathing in, I see myself as a child.

   Breathing out, I smile to the child that is still alive in me.

   Seeing myself as a child

   Smiling

8. Breathing in, I see the child in me as fragile, vulnerable, and having certain struggles and difficulties.

   Breathing out, I smile and embrace my inner child with my stable posture and mindful breathing.

Seeing the child fragile and vulnerable
Embracing

9. Breathing in, I recognize that the child's fragility, vulnerability, struggles, and difficulties continue to manifest in my daily life through my thoughts, speech, and bodily actions.
Breathing out, I smile and embrace my inner child with my stable posture and mindful breathing.

    Recognizing the child alive in me
    Embracing

10. Breathing in, I am aware that I am an adult now, with many positive conditions for practicing, healing, and transforming my inner child.
Breathing out, I feel hope and confidence in myself.

    Aware of positive conditions
    Feeling hopeful and confident

11. Breathing in, each mindful in-breath is joy and healing.
Breathing out, each mindful out-breath is joy and healing.

    Joy and healing
    In each breath

In the same sitting meditation session, after you have looked deeply into yourself as a child, you can move on to look deeply into your father as a child, and then into your mother as a child. Many teenagers have reported that this guided meditation helps them to see their parents as children, fragile and vulnerable, for the first time. Some may not be able to visualize this in the first session. Some adults cry or freeze when they meditate on their parents because so much pain arises; one should stay with the breathing and maintain a stable posture in this case. As you continue to practice this guided meditation a few times, you'll experience more empathy and understanding for your parents. For different reasons, you may also choose to look deeply into the child in yourself, in your father, and in your mother in separate sitting sessions. If this is the case, the first six steps are still the same; after that, use the following steps:

1. – 6. (as above)

7. Breathing in, I see my father/mother as a child.

Breathing out, I smile to the child that is still alive in my mother/ father.

> *Seeing my father/mother as a child*
> *Smiling*

8. Breathing in, I see the child in my father/mother as fragile and as having certain struggles and difficulties.

Breathing out, I smile and embrace the child in my father/mother with my stable posture and mindful breathing.

> *Seeing the child fragile, vulnerable, and struggling*
> *Embracing*

9. Breathing in, I recognize that the child's fragility, vulnerability, struggles, and difficulties continue to manifest in my daily life through my thoughts, speech, and bodily actions.

Breathing out, I smile and embrace the child in my father/mother in me with my stable posture and mindful breathing.

Recognizing the child of father/mother alive in me

Embracing

10. Breathing in, I am aware that I am an adult now, with many positive conditions to practice, heal, and transform my father's/mother's inner child in me.

Breathing out, I feel hope and confidence in myself.

Aware of positive conditions

Feeling hopeful and confident

11. Breathing in, each mindful in-breath is joy and healing.

Breathing out, each mindful out-breath is joy and healing.

Joy and healing

In each breath

COLLECTIVE ENERGY

As monastic practitioners, we live together in a community known as a Sangha. I live with my sisters twenty-four hours a day. Usually, we live in the same monastery for a few years, before moving to another sister monastery. The Plum Village monasteries all over the world are sister monasteries.

If you live with one person, and you can't bear it, imagine living with twenty women or sometimes two hundred women on the same monastery grounds! It can be quite crowded. There can be a lot of suffering to endure. Yet for the most part we're actually joyful and kind toward each other, because we aren't just women; we are also spiritual practitioners.

Most days we have two periods of sitting meditation. In the meditation hall, everyone sits together, and each person has a chance to learn how to look at his or her own cosmos quietly and practice deep listening and loving speech with oneself; this is the foundation for speaking and listening compassionately to another person.

Because we're sitting together in the same hall, everyone contributes to the collective energy, which in turn supports everyone else. Usually, I cannot sit by myself for two hours or even one hour. My mind will start to think: "Is it done yet? It must be time already." However, when I sit with the Sangha, I can sit for as long as the Sangha sits, and sometimes, such as in meetings, that can be for over three hours. Anchored in my breathing and in my body, I entrust myself to the collective energy of the Sangha. Whether we're sitting quietly or sitting in a Dharma talk or in a meeting, I dwell solidly in body and mind.

It is this collective energy that has enabled me to sit with my suffering from the very beginning of my monastic life. Up to and including the present time, I continue to take refuge in the collective energy of the Sangha in order to understand myself more deeply and to live in harmony with my sisters.

Living in community, I can see my habit energies and my difficulties by looking at myself as well as at my sisters. I am sincerely determined to transform and heal my habit energies and my suffering. I can still see myself getting upset or saying harsh words, but over the years, this happens less frequently and much more mildly than before.

Recognizing that my habit energies are deeply ingrained, I learn to be patient with myself. I learn to understand the workings of my mind. Thus, when I see somebody else behaving in a similar way, or even in a totally different way that is unskillful, I can understand his or her mind process.

The insight of interbeing also makes it possible for me to see myself in others. If somebody is unskillful, perhaps at another time I would have felt criticism or disappointment, but now I stop myself and recognize that I am not different from this person. Perhaps in the past I have done exactly the same thing. I may be doing the exact same thing right now, and that person's behavior helps me see my behavior, my speech, and my thinking more clearly. Even if I haven't done that particular unskillful thing in the past or in the present, it's still possible that in the future, when I'm in a certain situation, I'll behave the same way as that person.

This line of right thinking quiets my judgment and criticism of others, helping me to have more patience and to give them more support, time, and space to be themselves and to transform. Furthermore, it helps me to reflect upon myself and learn not to repeat the unskillful things that other people may do. Everyone can become a mirror image for me so that I may understand my own mind better, transform my habit energies, and gain insights that help me and that I can offer to others.

If we don't have direct experience with ourselves, we might still expect the other person to change. But that expectation is unrealistic because we aren't doing anything to help that person to transform. On the contrary, we burden that person additionally because of our harsh speech or impatient behaviors.

The insight of interbeing reminds us that each of us contains the whole cosmos, and the cosmos within each of us is not at all separate from that of any other.

If we want change, first of all we need to direct that energy inward. We must have a spiritual dimension in our lives with concrete daily practices to help us cultivate understanding and love in ourselves, so that we may truly live in harmony with our family and community and support them in their endeavors.

This is an ongoing process. It doesn't mean that we must become fully self-realized in order to live with other people and help them, but we do always have to come back and practice with ourselves.

It would be very helpful if the other person has the same practice and understands that we're trying our best. For example, our monastic brothers and sisters are aware that we are all sincere practitioners. However unskillful we may be with each other, we remind ourselves that we invest our lives in the practice and that we need each other in order to continue on the path.

FORGIVENESS

People often ask, "How can I forgive somebody when that person has hurt me so much?" This person may be somebody who raped us or betrayed us. This person may be our partner who said and did something so painful to us. This person may be our own child. This person may be ourself whom we've neglected and abused. How can we forgive?

Interbeing is a practice that allows us to forgive. When we can see, through the insight of interbeing, that "this is because that is," "this is in that," and "this is that," then we're able to forgive.

Forgiveness is not a kind of amnesia, a forgetting of the past. As long as our mind is intact, we remember our past experiences. Yet the insight and the practice of interbeing can help us heal these wounds from within. We realize that we have become the perpetrators of our own suffering. The other person might have been unskillful or unjust toward us at one time or during a certain period of years, but since that time we've continued that abusive pattern toward ourselves up and into the present.

One of my best friends said that her father always called her stupid whenever she was clumsy or did something wrong. When we were in college together, and every time she accidently dropped something, got a bad grade, or did something not so well, she would say aloud, "I'm so stupid! Stupid!"

With mindfulness, we recognize how we've repeatedly wounded ourselves, and slowly we learn to say, "I'm sorry. I don't want to do that to myself ever again." We learn to use loving speech and deep listening toward ourselves. If by chance we say, "I'm stupid," then we can gently correct it by saying, "I'm sorry. I didn't mean that." We breathe, smile, and relax that harsh thought and feeling.

Sometimes when I'm walking, I may accidently bang my hand or another part of my body on something like the edge of a table, and it's painful. I don't know when, maybe even before I became a nun, I learned to say, "I'm sorry" to the desk or to whatever it was that I accidently hit. Some people may kick or hit the thing that caused them pain, and they get more pain and anger as a result. The Buddha taught about the "second arrow." There is pain from the first arrow, but if we strike at the wound site with a second arrow, the pain will multiply. Thus, when we stop and say "I'm sorry" to the desk, we block the second arrow. We touch the wound and massage it tenderly; it is soothed, and no further pain is inflicted.

Similarly, when we recognize that we've been the perpetrators of our suffering and pain, we learn to say we're sorry toward ourselves, and we learn to look for ways to do things differently. Then we heal from the inside.

This is, because that is. Looking deeply, we see that the person who has hurt us has also suffered in his or her life. Someone might hurt a child, because he or she had been hurt as a child, or had witnessed other adults hurting children in that certain way. It may have been the only way the person had seen how children should be treated. Haunted by cruel and perverse images, the victim inadvertently rehearsed them and strengthened a particular neural pathway in his or her brain. The things we think will often manifest in our corresponding speech and bodily actions. Thus, unknowingly, the victim becomes the perpetrator.

Only from this revelation and breakthrough can we empathize with the other person, forgive him or her, and move forward with our lives. We too need our own forgiveness.

ATTENDING YOUR OWN FUNERAL

In our time, all over the world people commit suicide, most notably teenagers and young people in their late teens, twenties, and thirties. In an attempt to discourage this alarming trend, some businesses in Korea have made it possible for people to experience their own funerals. People can choose their own coffin and funeral clothing. They have a chance to write their living will and reflections. Then they come into the coffin, lie down, and experience the entire funeral ceremony done for them. They can even request to have the lid of the coffin closed for a while.

Most people going through this trial-death experience have reported that they felt strongly moved as they were writing their living will. It felt so real to them that some started to cry and tried to make peace with themselves and their loved ones.

The last words they wanted to write were often to their children, to their spouses, to people who had caused them suffering, or to those whose suffering they had caused. They wanted to apologize, to begin anew, and to forgive themselves and others.

While lying inside the coffin, many felt intense fear, even though they knew they could sit up and get out of it any time. Those who had the coffin lid closed down even felt panic.

Once these people stepped out of the coffin, they felt incredibly relieved. Life was wonderful and beautiful!

Perhaps we, too, have been in the trial coffin many times without being aware of it. Being in a destructive relationship, whether it's with ourself or with other people, can be like being in a coffin. If we're able to get out of it, we feel so fresh and alive. Yet if we don't know how to take care of our way of thinking, speaking, and behaving, we may return to our old habit energies, and in due time we're enclosed in the same or another coffin.

Mindfulness practices enable us to touch our everyday life deeply and to renew our relationships and interactions constantly. We can truly see a flower and not the category "flower." We can truly see our beloved in this very moment, and not through the lens of the past. It's like seeing the blue sky for the first time.

BLUE SKY

A retreat participant fell while he was playing Frisbee in the field in front of the nunnery. He was big like a football player, and he must have hurt his ankle badly, because he lay stretched out on the grass, moaning in pain. Sister Noble Truth said to him, "Smile. Look at the blue sky and smile!"

The man was confused. He was in so much pain, and he didn't understand why she told him to look at the blue sky and smile.

Another sister was also there, and she was afraid that this man would be hurt by Sister Noble Truth's comment. She tried to explain to him that it was our practice to touch the present moment. There is the pain, and there is also the blue sky.

Sister Noble Truth was standing behind this elder sister, and she kept poking her head out and telling him, "Smile. Look at the blue sky! This is a happy moment!"

Suddenly, he got it. He saw the blue sky and he laughed and laughed until the brothers came to take him to the hospital. It turned out to be a sprained ankle.

From then on, every time he passed by Sister Noble Truth, he would smile brightly or say to her, "Look at the blue sky," or "This is a happy moment!" Our friend was on crutches for a few weeks, but he was able to enjoy the blue sky and many happy moments with us.

Mindfulness practice helps us to see the blue sky even in the midst of an argument or difficult situation in a relationship. We learn to see each other as if we're seeing the blue sky for the first time. This provides space in us so we can cool down and—however difficult the relationship may be—we can remember our love for each other and the sincere efforts and dreams that we have shared together. That is our blue sky, reminding us that we need to return and take care of every moment.

The most important skill I've learned in my monastic life is to renew myself in every moment. This may take only a mindful breath, a mindful step, a smile, or a pause to look at a flower or the sky. Then I can be solid, spontaneous, and present for myself and for the blue sky, so that I can be that way for others and their difficulties.

A FALL WHILE JOGGING

I injured my ankle while jogging at Deer Park Monastery. I didn't dare tell my sisters what had really happened, out of fear that they would reproach me. I was jogging down toward the main gate. The road had been repaved recently, so it was smooth and beautiful. Blooming lilacs were everywhere. It was a gorgeous day. I was happily running from this side to the other side, zigzagging on the road. I was so happy that I ended up closing my eyes while running. That was how—right at the junction of the concrete road and the dirt road—I accidently went off the road, lost my balance, and fell down.

Once my brother Sonny asked me, "When you fall, do you look around?" "Why?" I asked. My brother replied, "I usually look around to see if people saw me falling."

I sat very still. A sharp, piercing pain went right through my body. I stayed with my in-breath and out-breath. I was aware of the waves of pain that rose and fell, rose and fell. I continued to sit very still and follow my breathing. I don't know how long I actually sat like that.

After a while the pain seemed to be less intense. Slowly and gently, I flexed and extended my ankle and rotated it side to side to see if it had been fractured. The movements were limited and painful, but possible.

I sat still and breathed some more. There I was, sitting on the side road, staying fully present for the pain. There was no fear or worry. I wasn't literally looking at the blue sky, but my mind was quiet and calm, and that was my blue sky. My blue sky was my breathing. My blue sky was the relaxation of my body. My blue sky was my awareness and embracing of the pain.

The pain subsided with time. Since it was possible that no one would be driving by for many hours, I risked standing up and then slowly walked back to the monastery. I was limping a little, but there wasn't that much pain. Later my ankle became very swollen and painful, so I had to immobilize it and massage it for many weeks with alcohol mixed with herbal medicine prepared by one of our elder sisters in the community.

FALLING OFF AN OAK TREE

I fell another time, at the end of our 2009–10 Winter Retreat. During the ten lazy days I practiced Noble Silence. One day, a group of our brothers and sisters went on a hike. Everybody was talking joyfully, but I maintained Noble Silence.

We came to our favorite oak tree. It was gigantic, with many branches as thick as trees themselves. As we had done before, each one of us would find a branch, climb up on it, and then lie on the branch and relax for a long while.

It was a day at the end of the winter. It was still cold and wet and there was moss growing on the branches. I wanted to reach a particular branch, but instead of climbing up the trunk to get to it, I tried to reach it from the ground. The branch was at eye level, so it wasn't possible to climb up onto it. Therefore, I tried to pull myself up, but the branch was so big around that I wasn't able to get a good grip. The first time I tried to pull myself up, it didn't work at all. The next time, I managed to get into the air for a moment. But because of my bad grip I wasn't able to use all my strength, and I fell backward. My back hit the ground and my lower back landed right on a log. In that moment I experienced an excruciating pain from my back and downward.

I lay very still, and I thought to myself that my spine could be injured, and that I was probably paralyzed right now. With that thought I didn't dare to move even one hair's breadth. I just lay very still with my back on the log and breathed. I breathed through the waves of pain. I lay there for a long time, so long that one brother on a nearby branch finally said, "Sister D, are you okay? Are you okay?"

I didn't respond. I just continued to breathe. Then the brother said to one of my sisters, "Sister, would you go down and see if something happened to Sister D? See if she's okay."

My sister climbed down from her branch and asked me, "Are you okay?" I didn't say anything. Eventually I slowly tried to move my leg and saw that I could move. I sat up quietly, and she gave her hand to me. I held her hand, stood up, and tried to take one step and then another. I was able to move but with much pain and effort.

Soon after that, we all left the tree together, but I continued to remain in Noble Silence. My brothers and sisters walked slowly enough that I lagged just a little behind. I was in severe pain for over a week, and I had to move with extreme care.

A few months later when we were going on another hike, somehow it was recalled that I had fallen from the tree that day. I told my brothers and sisters that I had been in severe pain and that in that moment I hadn't known whether I was paralyzed or not.

My brother asked, "Why didn't you say anything?" I replied, "Well, I was in Noble Silence." He said, "What? In that moment you were still keeping Noble Silence?"

I just smiled. I guess it was my stubbornness, which has helped me go through life. More than that, I was truly in Noble Silence, not with just my mouth, but also in my mind. My mind stayed with my breath and with my body, and I was calm and at ease. The physical pain was undoubtedly there, but the mental anxiety and suffering were not.

SUFFERING IS OPTIONAL

As spiritual practitioners, we train our mind to anchor itself in our breath and body in our daily lives. Whenever a situation arises, however pleasant or unpleasant it is, we already have the capacity and skills to dwell in this awareness, which enables us to go through the process as peacefully and calmly as possible. This is the foundation for a healthy future. Thus, we see that pain is inevitable, but suffering is truly optional.

In a moment of serious crisis or injury, the body can release large amounts of adrenaline. This enables a person to walk miles on a broken foot in order to seek help, or a mother to lift a car to save her child caught beneath it. The high surge of adrenaline blocks the pain and enables us to deal with the dangerous situation.

Through my own experiences, I have learned that in these traumatic moments, if we can come back to our breath and our body and relax, we can calm the waves of pain, and then our body no longer has to continue to secrete adrenaline into the bloodstream.

We sit still and stay calm, instead of being frightened and reactive. If we twist or move impulsively, we may make the injury worse, which in turn causes the release of more adrenaline. When so much adrenaline or cortisone is secreted, the body becomes exhausted afterward.

It's just like in an emergency room—when an attending physician calls for a Code Blue, everyone in the code team starts to run toward the patient's room and do everything they can to resuscitate or intubate the patient. The emergency room is entirely on alert to take care of this dire situation. Afterward the place looks like a battlefield. Things are thrown all over the floor. The air is taut with energy. Everybody has moved on to the next task, but their minds and bodies may still be trembling and shaken from the experience.

This may be the experience of our own body too after a crisis. Some people may be in a daze; others may sleep for days on end.

Unfortunately, sometimes we don't even allow ourselves to sleep and rest, so that the body has a chance to calm down and replenish itself, and the mind can process and heal from the trauma. Instead, the body will continue to go through the traumatic experience for a prolonged time, physiologically and psychologically. The damage comes not only from the psychological or physical injury itself, but also from the aftermath, the aftereffect of the adrenaline and the unresolved disturbance and fatigue of body and mind.

In post-traumatic stress disorder (PTSD), the person relives the experience over and over again, and the body goes through the physiological stress response as if the situation were actually happening. Thus, the traumatic event doesn't take place only once, but it is experienced every time the victim relives it. The resulting neural pathway may start as a faint trail, but with constant rehearsing, it becomes like a freeway, easily triggered by sights, sounds, smells, tastes, touch, or thoughts that are associated with the initial stressful event.

In this scenario, time doesn't heal. The ghost of the past dictates the present moment. Understanding this, we see the importance of how we choose to approach and go through a stressful situation. The process itself can actually determine the outcome, both short-term and long-term.

When I experienced the injury of my ankle, then my back, and then later on with Lyme disease, I went through it with mindfulness of my breathing and of my body. There was stability, peace, and relaxation. As a result, much energy was preserved in order to heal my body. Now when I recall these experiences, my body doesn't go through a physiological stress response. My memory of these events is not one of trauma.

SADNESS WAS HIS SICKNESS

I remember a patient who I met when I was doing an internship in Kenya. I asked this scrawny, elderly man, "What is your sickness?" He gently replied, "Sadness is my sickness. Sickness is my sadness."

His answer became a riddle to me. It stayed with me, and as I practiced more, I see that our body holds our sadness, our anger, and the traumatic experiences that we've gone through in life. Our body holds our pain and suffering.

In dualistic thinking, we think that the body is different from the mind. Yet in Western psychology we already have the concept of psychesoma. Psyche means the mind, and soma means the body. There are illnesses that we call psychosomatic. The root of the illness may be in the mind, but it manifests in the body.

For example, during the Killing Fields atrocities, Cambodian women witnessed their children being torn apart by the Khmer Rouge right in front of them. They witnessed their husbands being tortured and killed. The pain was so excruciating for them that afterward they became blind, even though when the doctors examined them, their optic nerves were intact and their occipital lobes were also intact. Yet they could not see.

These women were psychologically blind. Their mind shut down their vision because it couldn't bear to look and see anymore. This is a psychosomatic illness—it's a pain of the mind that manifests in the body. There are many psychosomatic illnesses widely recognized in Western psychology and medicine.

With our awareness that the body's pain and suffering is rooted in the mind, we need to pay attention to the pain instead of simply numbing it with medication or using entertainment to forget it. Looking deeply into the pain, we can find the roots of our suffering. It may be rooted in the mind, in certain worries, anxieties, fears, and traumas that we haven't yet resolved. Yet it manifests in the body, and because the body is something tangible, we're able to touch it, see it, hear it, feel it, and perceive it.

This is useful, because we can work with our suffering by coming back to befriend our own body, showing affection and love toward it. The process of healing can begin in the body, and in that process, we discover the deeper roots of our suffering in the mind.

When the body is calmed and soothed, the mind also becomes calmer and more soothed, and it will unfold itself to us more clearly. This is the interbeing nature of body and mind. Recognition of the pain and suffering leads us to the understanding of its root, which in turn shows us the way to take care of it and to cultivate true love and peace.

SKY OF STARS

Two years into my monastic life, I had an epiphany while I was lying on my bed box one day. Each of us has a bed box that's knee high and barely longer than my five-foot, six-inch body. It has two flat lids on which we sleep, and we put all of our belongings inside it.

I was staying on the second floor of the Purple Cloud Hall in New Hamlet, and there was a skylight in our room. As I was lying on the bed box, I looked out the skylight window and saw some stars. I was deeply happy and content to look at those stars.

Then a thought arose in my mind, "I wish I could stay in this room for a few years so I can enjoy this beautiful view." Soon a second thought came to me, "Out there the sky is full of stars. Why do I want to live in this room content to only see a few stars?"

This simple thought has become a guiding light for me. Sometimes I may feel comfortable or justified in thinking a certain way about myself or about somebody else. But then I also remind myself that I can be so much more free, happy, and at peace if I open my heart, step out of this confined space, and go into the open sky where I can see that my brothers and sisters are myself, that I am them, and that we are all the continuations of our Teacher, of the Buddha, of this life, and that we can rejoice in whatever we can offer to each other and to the world without feeling superior or inferior, without grasping or aversion.

REACTION TIME

Even though I studied medicine, I would never consider myself a scientific or technologically oriented person. I know how to use the computer just well enough to type and write articles, poems, and songs. One time, I was trying to send a fax, but I didn't know how to operate the machine. An elder sister, who was in the office at the time, had great technical skills. She patiently showed me how to use the machine, but I'd forgotten by the next time, so she became irritated. She said, "And you are a doctor?"

I just smiled brightly. I didn't feel bad at all in that moment. Had I been a technology wizard, I might not have become a nun.

There is something simple about me, and the monastic practice allows me to be happily simple. If someone had said that to me before I'd ordained, maybe I would have felt offended or sad. Interestingly, the capacity to be in the present moment helps me to take what is happening as an isolated event, without tagging interpretations and judgments onto it.

Often when something happens, I find myself taking it in, but not thinking much about it or reacting to it. Sometime later, I may regret not having said something clever in response. Then I smile to myself, feeling happy that I could simply be there for the person or the situation as it was.

CLEANING TOILETS

At Deer Park Monastery, we held at least one retreat a month; and during my seven years living there, I volunteered to clean toilets during most of those retreats. After a while, I didn't even need to volunteer because the organizing teams would assign me that task automatically; they knew that I was willing to do it.

I would lead a family that helped me with this task. If there were teenagers in the retreat, I would lead them in our Dharma sharing group, and during the working period we would clean toilets. Some teens found it repugnant at first, but most of them would show up daily to help.

In the Vietnamese-language retreats, I also led the Dharma discussion family in cleaning toilets. One lay friend got offended. She said she was always happy to be in my family for Dharma sharing, but then she had to clean toilets, year after year.

Personally, I don't have a problem with it. I never think that since I'm a doctor, I shouldn't have to clean toilets. In fact, early in my monastic life I saw that cleaning toilets is as important as giving Dharma talks. It has trained me to be more humble and inclusive.

As I'm cleaning the toilet, I recite the Heart of Perfect Understanding Sutra: "All dharmas are marked with emptiness. They are neither produced nor destroyed, neither defiled nor immaculate, neither increasing nor decreasing." The toilet is a mirror of my mind, and the art of cleaning the toilet is analogous to the art of cleaning my mind.

Without fail, every time I would clean the toilet, I would also use it. It is clean, and I am the first one to benefit from it. Similarly, as we transform our own suffering, we are the first one to benefit from that and then others will be able to benefit from it as well. Whatever we do is wonderfully important, whether others recognize our work or not. We may be working alone and silently, but deep joy arises because we know that we are present for ourself and we are purifying our mind.

I have learned to be willing to take on any kind of job, to see the importance in everything I do—in walking, in sitting, in using the toilet, whether there are people around me or not, and whether it is daytime or nighttime. When I wake up in the middle of the night, I'm the only one to see myself. As long as I have mindfulness, I can be present and look at myself with all honesty. There is no discrimination or distinction in this practice, and it gives me peace throughout the day and night. This energy of mindfulness is what I return to moment after moment. It is to be my own soul mate.

I have half jokingly said to people that in my life I have been passionate about many things, including people, animals, plants, and minerals. These different kinds of passion come and go, but as a monastic practitioner for almost fifteen years now, I have never doubted the Dharma. I have never felt that the Dharma isn't effective or interesting. Practicing the Dharma has given me the reason to live. I can touch joy and peace in every moment that I'm mindful, and even if the moment is difficult, even if it's full of despair and sadness, the energy of mindfulness helps me to embrace that despair and sadness; I can still smile while tears are streaming down.

MUD IN LOTUS

When we have pain, physical or mental, we tend to look for a way to avoid it. To treat physical pain, we often turn to medication to numb or resolve it. For mental pain, we seek adventures, entertainment, conversations, relationships, food, drugs, and career in order not to face our suffering.

Interestingly, if we look deeply into our body, deep teaching is present there. When the body is in trouble, sensory nerves are innervated and we experience pain. These sensations of pain alert us that the body is in trouble. If we couldn't experience pain, we wouldn't be aware that the body is injured. We wouldn't feel any urgency to take care of the wound.

Consider people with leprosy or Hansen's disease. The bacteria of leprosy look very much like the bacteria of tuberculosis, they're what are called acid-fast bacilli. These bacteria live in the sensory nerves of the affected person and damage them, especially the nerves in the distal limbs like the hands and the feet.

Normally, if we hit our hand on a table or other hard object, we feel pain and immediately pull our hand back. We learn to move about skillfully in order not to hit our hands and limbs on hard things, and when they're hurt, we tend to them right away. People with leprosy don't feel pain when they accidentally hit their hands on something hard. Consequently, they don't consciously avoid hitting hard things, and so their skin is damaged repeatedly, which can often lead to infection. Without pain, they're not motivated to take care of the wound or infection promptly. The infection spreads inward from the skin to the muscles and even to the bones. After a while, the fingers have to be amputated in order to save the rest of the limb or to prevent sepsis, by which the infection spreads systemically via the bloodstream.

It becomes a vicious cycle: people with leprosy have damaged sensory nerves, they feel no pain, so they don't take good care of their wounds and, as a result, their limbs and bodies become further damaged and deformed.

Thus, pain is a mechanism that motivates us to take care of ourselves. When animals are injured, they immediately find a quiet, secluded area where they can lie down and rest. They may look for some leaves that have medicinal value to treat their wound. They don't chase after animals for food or for mating, but instead, they tend to their wound. They lie still, resting and possibly sleeping, until their body heals itself.

In our modern times, we've forgotten our capacity to heal. We actually forget that pain is a protective mechanism. When we have pain, instead of listening to it so we can understand the injury that caused it and we can tend to it appropriately, we find ways to suppress the pain and to forget about it. That's why physical and mental pain continues to infest us and to spread deeper and wider.

As practitioners, we learn to see the interbeing nature of pain, which is a sign of ill-being, and health, which is a sign of well-being. There is an interbeing relationship between illness and wellness, between pain and non-pain, between suffering and happiness. We learn to be there for the pain and even to "enjoy" it while it is there. Pain can be a friend and a teacher through which we discover ourselves.

In Vietnamese and Buddhist culture, we use the image of the lotus flower to illustrate this. The lotus flower grows beautifully above the surface of the water. It usually has a pinkish color mixed with white, and it has a sweet, spicy fragrance.

In the old days, people would row a small boat out on the lotus pond in the late afternoon or early evening while the lotus petals were still open. They would place a tiny bag of tea on the stamen of each flower. In the evening, the petals would close, enfolding the tea inside the flower, and the tea would absorb the fragrance of the lotus throughout the night. In the morning, when the petals opened up, the people would row back out to the lotus flowers and pick up their bags of tea. They knew the art and the leisure of making tea with lotus fragrance and enjoying it.

The Buddha is often portrayed sitting on a lotus throne. The Buddha doesn't sit on a golden throne but simply on a lotus flower. The lotus exudes elegance, beauty, and wholesomeness, and when we look closely we see that the lotus has come from mud. The lotus grows only in mud where its roots can penetrate deeply. From there, the stem will push upward through the water and above the surface. At first it may look like the tip of a brand-new calligraphy brush that's breaking through the surface. But once it's slightly above the surface of the water the tip slowly grows bigger and the petals open.

The lotus is elegant and fragrant, but it comes from mud, which is dark and pungent. The mud is not only in the pond, where it continues to provide nutrients to the thriving lotus, but the mud is also present in every fiber of the plant. So the lotus is made from non-lotus elements, including water, sunshine, and mud. The mud is absolutely essential to the manifestation of the lotus. This is the interbeing nature of the mud and the lotus, which becomes the symbolic place of peace and stability for the Buddha.

I believe it was during the US Tour of 2007, when we were at Deer Park Monastery, that Thay gave me a written request from a retreatant, who wanted Thay to write a calligraphy for him. It read something like: If there is not the mud of suffering and ignorance, there could not be the lotus of true happiness and enlightenment. It was a long, winding sentence. Thay asked if I could shorten it. I focused on the piece of paper, breathing for a while. Then I looked up at Thay and simply said, "No mud. No lotus." Just that, and Thay smiled.

Suffering is an element of the Four Noble Truths, because when there's an understanding of suffering, this leads to the way out of suffering and into happiness. Without understanding, there's nothing noble about suffering. Mud is just mud, sticky and stinky.

True happiness derives from a deep understanding of our suffering and of the workings of our mind. It isn't the happiness that most of us are acquainted with. It isn't the kind of happiness that we feel when we eat a bar of chocolate, enjoy the taste, and get a sugar high. It isn't the happiness that makes us become verbose or excited in our thoughts, speech, or bodily actions. It isn't the happiness we feel when we're high on drugs, or when we're falling in love with someone. These forms of happiness that most of us are acquainted with come and go quickly, and they're usually associated with forgetfulness and latent suffering.

During one of our retreats at the YMCA of the Rockies, a thirteen-year-old boy shared that as he was trying to eat a chocolate chip cookie slowly that day, he'd discovered that it tasted like cardboard! He loved to eat that kind of cookie, but he realized that they were only good because he always ate them quickly.

On the contrary, the happiness that we touch when the mind is one with the body and the present moment, is quiet, calm, bright, light, and at the same time, enduring. It's more like when we eat a piece of broccoli or carrot slowly and its texture and sweetness dissolve on our tongue. This sweetness is calming to our mind. We're aware that its nourishing effect is long-lasting.

Mindfulness is like the moonlight that we can use to shine onto our suffering. We realize that suffering is not as menacing or threatening as we may have perceived it to be all of our lives. With the gentle moonlight, we can sit quietly and embrace suffering with our mindful breathing and upright, stable posture.

We may still cry, but we're crying with our suffering, not because of it. We may talk to our suffering as we would talk to a friend or to our own child. We know how to massage the pain, relax and soften it with mindful breathing in and out, cradling it like a child. Suffering will blossom into insight, acceptance, and forgiveness, as we understand its roots and feel great empathy toward ourselves.

We can discover that our suffering isn't ours alone. Often we suffer not only because of a painful situation but also because we feel that we're the only ones who are suffering. Embracing suffering with tenderness, our mindfulness is already a comforting companion that gives us the ability to listen deeply to ourselves, to be our own soul mates who can be there to remember, know, understand, and heal our own suffering.

In this process, we also discover that the sources of our suffering are not only within us. They have come from our parents, ancestors, society, and from innumerable other factors. We don't have to hold onto our suffering or bear it all by ourselves. We can call on our parents and our ancestors to help us hold it. We transform this suffering not only for ourselves but for them as well.

Understanding our own suffering will help us touch the suffering in others and alleviate it.

THE CRYING LITTLE GIRL

Recently when we held a retreat for families, a child was crying uncontrollably and three adults were trying to soothe her. I happened to walk by so I asked, "What's wrong, my child? What's wrong?" Apparently the other children had left her out of an activity.

I tried to pick her up. She was about eight years old and a bit heavy for me, but I picked her up anyway and embraced her in my arms. I said, "Shush, quiet down my child. It's okay. It's okay."

She was still crying and I told her, "Look at the blue sky! Look, isn't that so beautiful?" She looked up and even though she still wanted to cry, the moment she looked at the blue sky she couldn't cry anymore. I said, "Look at that. You see, even though you're in pain, the blue sky is still beautiful, and life is still beautiful. Will you always remember this?"

She wiped the last of her teardrops and nodded her head. I put her down and then some of her friends came. They all had learned the practice of Beginning Anew, so they hugged her and gave her the flowers they had just collected in order to make peace with her. Then they all held hands and walked away together joyfully.

Another mother and her child were still there. The mother said to her child, "You have suffered exclusion many times. I don't understand why, when you saw her suffering like that, you didn't help her. Why is that?"

The child replied, "I was feeling left out myself!" as she stomped away. I told the mother, "You know, suffering on its own doesn't bring empathy. It can make people ruthless. It can make people believe, 'I have suffered; you don't know anything about suffering, and you should suffer some.'"

The mother was shocked and said, "That's cruel!"

I told her, "That's right. It's only the understanding of our own suffering that will help us connect with other people, understand them in turn, and want to help them. Please talk to your child and help her explore her feelings so that she understands what she feels when she's left out. When she understands that and she learns ways not to feel left out, then she can help other people."

USING THE BODY FOR REVENGE

In November 2005, I went to Prajna Monastery in Vietnam to help train about two hundred young nuns and aspirants. I met a young woman in her early twenties, who had been staying with the sisters for almost a year, but she wasn't allowed to ordain yet because she had many problems. She told me that as a child, she had lived with her parents in a mountainous area. Her parents were neighbors with two young men who were brothers. Since the time she was ten years old, these two brothers took turns coming to her house when her parents were away working, taking her out into the field, and raping her. She had never dared to say anything to her parents.

When she was fifteen, she was sent to Saigon to go to school. She was in so much pain and anger that she decided to take revenge. She would have sexual relationships with married men. She would keep their love letters or she would take photographs of them having sexual intercourse with her, but without her face showing, and then she would send their letters and photographs to their wives in order to destroy their families. That was her way of taking revenge on men.

When Thay went back to Vietnam in the beginning of 2005, she heard about Thay and went to one of his retreats. Her heart was opened, and she didn't want to continue in her way of revenge anymore. She followed the monastics to Hue in central Vietnam and asked permission to stay and become an aspirant. She was so stubborn and also had a strong tendency to be attracted and attached to the sisters, so they were cautious with her. They allowed her to continue to stay with them, but they didn't dare to ordain her. Very often this young woman wouldn't be able to sleep at night, because she had severe bouts of abdominal pain. I was practicing Noble Silence on our Lazy Mondays, and she would come to me at ten o'clock on a Sunday night to try to talk to me. She said, "I know you'll be practicing Noble Silence tomorrow, but you know how I fear these episodes of abdominal pain and this insomnia." I told her, "Talking with me now won't change your situation. You've been having insomnia and abdominal pains for many years. You know the reason why. Breathe with them." I wasn't being cruel. I knew it was also something she used to get attention from the sisters. At first she got very angry with me and stomped away. Later she came around again to talk to me. I asked her, "Do you know why I wouldn't talk to you that night?" She said, "I know you want me to take care of this. You want me to use the practice to take care of my pain instead of depending on the sisters."

Every moment our cells are sloughing off and regenerating. It's said that every seven years we have a completely renewed body. Yet the pain and suffering continue, because our way of thinking about the past is the same. Women with a history of sexual abuse may later have boyfriends or husbands, but they continue to look at their body and at sex in a very negative way, which inadvertently perpetuates the abuse and the suffering. Furthermore, they transmit this negative attitude and view to their children, who will repeat the suffering. Therefore, to take care of our mind and our body is to heal them simultaneously. The mind is in the body, and it's reflected in what's going on in the body; the body is in the mind, and it reflects the pain or the healing of the mind.

SMILING TO BROWN SPOTS

I loved my grandmother who was there for me from the time I was born. Consequently, when I saw elderly people, I saw my grandmother in them, and I had a natural affection for them. Yet the thought that I would be old like that one day never crossed my mind. Now as I begin to grow older, I start to think about it more. Four years ago I saw the first brown spot on my hand, and it remained the only spot on my hand for three years. Then I got sick, and sometimes four brown spots can appear in a week! Since then, when I hold older people's hands, I become much more aware of the brown spots on their hands, and I give rise to the awareness that my hand will one day be like that. Maybe it will take place sooner than I wish. I see myself in them more concretely than ever.

Most of us don't think about sickness, aging, and death, until it arrives at our door. The truth is that this process takes place from the moment of our conception. An autopsy on a ten-year-old child reveals that there's already cholesterol buildup in the blood vessels. This buildup of fat in the blood vessels will attract calcium deposits, which cause the wall of the vessel to become thickened and rigid; this is known as atherosclerosis. As a result, the blood vessels will be less malleable and flexible, and that's a setup for high blood pressure and heart disease.

Don't think that sickness, old age, and death are very far away. They are already there, even if you're only twelve or thirteen years old. Look at the skin of young children; there are already blemishes, sunspots, and freckles. We play in the sun all day long without wearing a hat. I lived in Arizona for eight years, and I wore hats only as a fashion statement. All the college students around me were into suntanning, and no one told me that I should do my best to protect my skin. Instead of wearing sunblock, we wore suntan lotion. I learned later that when the skin gets tanned, it means our skin cells are damaged and they are secreting melanin to repair the cells. So this tan color is but an early sign of injury and illness. Again and again the skin cells try to repair themselves, but once we're in our thirties, forties, and fifties, the repairing process is weaker. When we're sick, new brown spots can just pop up literally every day. I was in dismay to see a big spot on my face one morning, which I hadn't seen the day before.

Aging is a natural process that takes place all the time. Nature reflects this clearly. However young the leaves may be, there already are holes in them. An apple, so delicious and shiny, also has spots and defects. Other fruits, too, are full of brown marks. Aging takes place from the time of conception so that our body can form and grow. Cells constantly die and regenerate. Aging is a part of life, but when we spend most of our time inside concrete walls, busy on the computer or talking on the phone, we aren't in touch with this process taking place in ourselves and all around us. We take for granted our youth and our good health, until an illness seems to intrude out of nowhere, and we're stricken with fear and terror.

Living closely with nature enables us to be in touch with impermanence, to reflect and apply to ourselves what we've observed in nature, and to transform our avoidance and fear of aging and death.

In the light of interbeing, we see that sickness, aging, and death are already present throughout our lifetime, and not just when we're old. When we have this insight, we appreciate life more deeply, we take good care of it, but we also learn not to cling to it. People are so afraid of death because they haven't lived fully. They haven't known what life is. That's why they cling to it at the last minute. Those who learn to know themselves, master themselves, and live their lives deeply and fully in each moment won't be afraid of death. They can smile to whatever is coming.

In our practice, we learn to smile often, whether or not we're happy. It's nice to smile when you're happy, but it's also important to cultivate a capacity to smile to all situations. When anger arises, instead of looking angry, just smile. When hurt hurls in, instead of looking hurt, just smile. This is a practice of nonfear toward anger and hurt. People have asked me, "Sister D, are you very happy? You must be very happy because you smile all the time." I tell them that I'm happy sometimes, but most of the time I'm smiling to my own crooked thoughts.

At night when I lie down on my bed box, I give rise to the thought that I may not wake up the next day. I'm forty-five years old and, as I review my day, I know that I have done my best to live mindfully, to be kind in my thoughts, speech, and bodily actions. I forgive my own unskillfulness. So if I don't wake up tomorrow, I can accept it. Then I smile and follow my breathing until I fall asleep. This is how I cultivate nonfear in my daily life. Nonfear is a great power. It's the power of love for ourselves and for others. We love not because we're needy, lonely, or don't know what to do with ourselves, so that we find another lonely, restless person to match up with and we get exponentially more lonely, restless, and confused. We love because we've learned to touch our liberated self, and we have understanding and nonfear to share with others.

Chapter Two

FRIENDSHIP

As monks and nuns, we close many doors.
But one door we have to keep open—that is the door of being human.

Maitri is the second Immeasurable Mind of Love (after upeksha, inter-being). It's a Sanskrit word that has been translated into English as "loving kindness."

The word "maitri" has its root in the word "mitra," which means friend. Therefore, Thay has suggested that we should retranslate maitri as "friendship, fraternity, brotherhood, or sisterhood."

In this light, we can translate maitri as friendship or kinship. Kinship means a relationship to somebody in your family, or a feeling of connectedness to somebody. In the Vietnamese language and culture, kinship is a deep and wide relationship between the people in the same biological family, as well as in the entire human family.

For example, in a family of blood-related brothers and sisters, siblings born earlier than ourselves are referred to as "older brothers" and "older sisters," not as "you" like in English. Because of this tradition, my brother Sonny always refers to me as "elder sister" in English. One time his American friend asked him, "Why do you call her 'sister?'" My brother innocently replied, "Because she is my sister!"

We always refer to ourselves in terms of our relationship to somebody. Therefore, if a stranger walks into someone's house, he can tell right away how people are related by listening to how they refer to themselves and to each other.

In a marital relationship, the husband is also referred to as an older brother, *anh*, and the wife is referred to as a younger sister, *em*. This is true in a dating relationship as well. In a patriarchal society, men are supposed to be the elders, providing shelter and protection to the family, so they are referred to as elder brothers.

In a social context, even when you first meet somebody, you will gauge to see if that person is older or younger than you. If the person is much older, you can refer to that person as a grandparent, uncle, or auntie, and you refer to yourself as the child of that person, *con*.

Therefore, it's embedded in Vietnamese as well as in many other languages that we see each other as relatives in the same greater human family and that we are all connected. We see ourselves in relationship to others; we see what our roles are in relation to them, and we behave accordingly.

This relatedness also extends to animals, and they are referred to as our children. All the animals have the word "con" in front of their names, and "con" literally means "child." For example, a cat is called *con meo*, or child cat. The dog is *con cho*. The fish is *con ca*.

Once while I was standing next to Thay as we were looking at an open field, he said to me gently, "Not only are the monks and nuns your brothers and sisters, but the dogs and the cats are also your brothers, sisters, and children. They also need you to help them cross to the other shore." To be honest, I didn't know exactly what Thay meant, but it was such a unique statement, that it has stayed with me all of these years. Gradually, I have come to understand that my practice is not just for myself, but for all of my family members in the human, animal, plant, and mineral realms. When my mind is peaceful and loving, there's no discrimination and judgment toward them. Helping to preserve and protect them become natural actions in my daily life.

Love is often directed toward an object outside us—a person, an animal, or a thing. Because that object is outside us, it's thought of as a possession: "This is my wife. This is my dog. This is my house." There's the "I" and the "you." This attitude of possessiveness can result in a lot of suffering. When a romantic relationship is going well, then we stay together; but if it isn't going well then we can just discard it.

A couple can easily divorce when they no longer want to have anything to do with each other. In the United States, more than sixty percent of marriages end in divorce. Most people believe that once they're divorced, they'll have nothing to do with each other anymore. The truth is that all the years and all the experiences that you have shared together continue to affect who you are and who your children will become. When you walk away from each other in anger and resentment, the suffering and bitterness keep escalating because you continue to think and argue with each other in your own minds. You may want your children to sever the communication with their father or mother, but that only causes your children to be more torn, confused, and lost. The mother and father who are present in every cell of their children's bodies become the target of reproach and rejection, and so many children grow up feeling hateful not only toward their parents but also toward themselves.

If we recognize each other as brothers and sisters, parents and children of each other, we will never think that we can completely sever our relationship. We will learn to take care of each other whether we're together or separated.

This kind of relatedness also extends to our own body. We can learn to treat our own body with love and reverence. Our body is our own kin, and we can befriend it. Most of us are so busy pursuing our careers and ambitions that we often don't even remember that we have a body. We can sit at the computer for eight hours straight and completely forget about this body. We suppress the need to use the restroom, we forget to eat, we forget our need to get up and move around, and we forget to rest.

If you want to love somebody, to have a friendship and kinship with that person, you must be able to experience all this in yourself first. Who will live with you twenty-four hours a day and for as long as you are still breathing? Who will be this constant and loyal companion—who but your own body?

In practicing maitri, we learn to direct love inward, cultivating friendship and kinship toward our own body and mind, listening and attending to our own needs, joys, and suffering.

In the Vietnamese culture, husband and wife are taught to behave and respect each other as new friends or as guests. They shouldn't change their clothes in front of each other. They should address each other appropriately. When people have known each other for a long time, they tend to become too casual toward each other. We're no longer careful with our words, and our speech can become harsh, rude, critical, judgmental, and disrespectful. We no longer listen to one another; as soon as the other person begins to speak, we've already assumed we know what he or she is going to talk about. The practice of seeing each other as new friends or guests helps us to remain cordial, respectful, and dignified toward ourselves and each other. The practice of loving speech and deep listening enables us to keep communication open and to continue to discover ourselves and one another anew, constantly growing and changing.

When I wake up in the morning, I give myself time to get acquainted with myself. I touch my shaven head to remind myself that I am a monastic practitioner and that I have another day to live in peace and harmony with myself. I massage my face, acknowledging my eyes and giving thanks to my eyes, acknowledging my nose and giving thanks to my nose, and so on. I am awakened to the fact that my sense organs are still intact, and this awareness fills me with gratitude and hope. I massage my chest, being aware of my lungs and my heart, and then I massage my abdomen, my back, my arms and legs. I refer to my body as my younger sister or my child. Sometimes I refer to myself as a child to my body. As I massage my body part-by-part, I become more alert and oriented, and I feel connected to my own body.

This practice also helps me to detect pain and tension that may exist in parts of my body. Without this awareness, pain and tension build up over the days, weeks, or years, and then they manifest themselves as physical or mental illness.

For example, somebody who has to think a lot may develop headaches. Somebody who is often depressed may manifest that as general malaise, lethargy, weakness, or chest pain. Somebody who smokes may end up with problems like chronic coughing, emphysema, pulmonary hypertension, or lung cancer.

As you befriend your body, you will recognize what a miracle it is, how it functions so diligently and harmoniously in order to make your life possible. You will realize that your body is bearing the physical pain, mental pain, and traumas of your life. Your body is marked by these experiences and burdened by them. This realization will give rise to empathy and gratitude to your own body. So often, I say to my body, "I have been unskillful. Please help me to take better care of you. Please help me embrace this pain and understand how it has come about. Please help me to take care of this pain, to heal and to transform it."

BLADDER CONTRACTING

In medical school, I went to see a doctor on campus about my abnormal urinary frequency. On my next visit the doctor said, "You know, I went to see a movie with my girlfriend the other day and suddenly I realized

I didn't have to go to the restroom halfway through. I remembered you said that even during a movie you would have to go at least once or twice, and I felt happy that I didn't have to miss the movie." I was embarrassed because this doctor went to a movie with his girlfriend and thought about my urinary problem. This incident helps me remember that I had this problem way back then.

In my monastic life, I have developed severe low blood pressure, Lyme disease, and then diabetes. As a result, my problem with urinary frequency has worsened. When I had symptomatic low blood pressure at Deer Park Monastery, with my systolic blood pressure in the eighties and diastolic blood pressure in the sixties, I would urinate about thirty times a day and five to seven times a night. It was exhausting. Sometimes when I had a room all to myself, I would keep a pot in the room, so I didn't have to walk down the stairway outside to get to the restroom. That walk would make me feel wide awake, so that it took me sometimes a half hour to fall back asleep, and then I'd have to wake up and use the restroom again.

I never knew why I had this problem. I never questioned how it came about. Then, just about five years ago, I had a vivid dream. In the dream, I was sitting on a sidewalk, and suddenly the memory of the sexual abuse I experienced as a child arose in my mind. At one point, I was holding up my own bladder in my hand, at eye level, and it was contracting randomly. It was like a heart in fibrillation or a bag full of worms moving chaotically about with no strength or unifying force.

The next morning during sitting meditation, for the first time I made the connection, that I had developed urinary frequency as a result of childhood sexual trauma. Within the week, I decided to go to a Chinese herbal doctor. He drew a picture of my bladder and explained to me in his broken English that at the funnel end of the bladder, the muscles were oversensitive and overstimulated, so it triggered the urge to empty itself before it was actually full. Otherwise, my kidneys and bladder were normal. Remembering my dream and what the herbal doctor said, I practiced visualizing my bladder stretching and contracting slowly, steadily, and synchronously. It was impossible at first, and then it became easier and more natural.

People carry their pain in different places. Some people carry it in their head and have headaches. Some people carry it in the chest and feel chest pain or shortness of breath. Other people develop skin problems. Women with a history of sexual abuse usually carry it in their abdominal organs, especially in the bladder, uterus, or digestive system. I have discovered that I carry my pain in my bladder, and every time I feel sick, weak, or nervous, when I go to sleep, or before I go somewhere, my bladder becomes hypersensitive and hyperactivated.

It all originated from a wounded child who didn't know how to express her pain or how to take care of her confusion and shame. The fear and pain were experienced in the bladder, weakening it and impairing it over time.

When you're young, the symptoms aren't obvious and they can be masked. As you grow older, you become weaker and contract certain illnesses, and the weakened parts will become weaker and more debilitating. If you tend to put pressure unevenly on one side of a foot, then the shoe on that foot becomes unevenly worn. Eventually, both shoes may have to be discarded just because the one part that you keep rubbing is so worn out. It is the same in our body.

To befriend our body is to recognize the kinship we have with it and to care for its joy as well as its suffering and pain. I have learned to be much more patient with myself every time I use the restroom. It is no longer different from doing sitting meditation in the meditation hall. Before I enter the bathroom, I knock on the door slowly three times, even if the door is open and no one is inside. This gives me a moment of stopping before I make a transition from the outside to the inside. I usually clean the toilet before I use it, silently reciting the gatha, the poem, for cleaning bathrooms:

> How wonderful it is
> to scrub and clean!
> Day by day,
> my heart and mind grow clearer.

Then as I sit down on the toilet, I recite:

> Sitting here
> is like sitting under a Bodhi tree.
> My body is mindfulness itself,
> free from all distraction.

I give myself time to breathe and relax my body, avoiding putting too much mental or physical pressure on the bladder or colon to empty quickly. Sitting upright and at ease, I recite "The Eight Realizations of the Great Beings" in Sino-Vietnamese, which I had memorized by heart, or the gatha for using the toilet:

> Defiled or immaculate, increasing or decreasing—
> these concepts exist only in our mind.
> The reality of interbeing
> is unsurpassed.

I give my body the time and space it needs to take care of me. Sometimes I put my hands gently on my abdomen, massaging it and sending the energy of love to my own body after I have gone to the restroom four times already in the night. "Thank you for trying," I tell my body. Frustration and despair do arise, but I breathe to calm these feelings so as not to worsen the situation. I am aware that it isn't my body's fault, and my body only needs love and empathy in order to heal. Instead of releasing more stress hormones, I send messages that are calming and loving so that mind and body may remain in oneness. I also practice certain qigong movements that can strengthen the kidneys and bladder and help them heal.

This relationship we develop with our own body is most important and most concrete in true love.

We tend to neglect or sacrifice our body in the pursuit of outside objects, and this behavior may have its root in the evolution of our ancestors—human, animal, plant, and mineral. Plants may not have a high level of consciousness, but they have the basic survival instinct. Plants will direct themselves toward the sun, known as phototaxis, as is shown in sunflowers. Certain plants will also move toward certain chemicals in the ground; this is known as chemotaxis. Another important survival strategy is to move toward a water source, roots digging deep and spreading far into the ground.

Reptiles have the brain stem and spinal cord that regulate heart rate, breathing rate, and also the fight-flight-freeze response. Animals' main behaviors are looking out for predators to avoid and for prey to feed themselves. When a sense of self began to develop in the limbic brain of the mammals, the need to ensure the confirmation and the survival of the self also formed, and so animals fight for territories, for mates, and for their offspring. All of these survival instincts continued to drive the *Homo erectus* and then the *Homo sapiens* of today.

However, during over two million years of evolution, humans have also developed the cortical brain, notably the frontal and prefrontal cortex, where higher cognitive functions reside, such as language, empathy, self-inhibition and self-awareness.

A cat can be aware of a mouse and maneuver instinctively to catch it, but the cat isn't aware of its own bodily movements or its feelings of excitement and anticipation. A human being, on the other hand, has the innate capacity to be aware of objects outside of her and, at the same time, of her own body, feelings, and thoughts.

Unfortunately, we don't often use this capacity of self-awareness in our daily lives. Like our animal ancestors, we're more aware of the objects outside of us. These outside objects may be our computers, our projects, the degrees we're working toward, or someone we're pursuing.

Meanwhile, the awareness we have of our own breathing, our own steps, the tension and pain in our body, the feelings of sadness, jealousy, or discrimination that we're experiencing in the present moment, may be minimal. That's why it's important to cultivate mindfulness of breathing, of walking, of our own body, so that we can be more self-aware and take better care of ourselves. Self-awareness and true love start with the body, because the body is the most concrete part of us, the part that we can see, hear, smell, taste, touch, and perceive.

It may have taken over two million years for *Homo erectus* to become *Homo sapiens*, but it takes only one mindful breath or one mindful step for the *Homo sapiens* to become "Homo conscious."

LOVING UTERUS

Another organ I have practiced to make peace with is the uterus. This practice is to acknowledge my unskillfulness, to begin anew with my own organs, and to ask my body to help me take better care of them.

At Deer Park Monastery, I developed low blood pressure and finally went to see a Chinese herbal doctor. At one point he told me that perhaps I was experiencing early perimenopausal symptoms because of my illness. He asked me how old my mother was when she went through menopause. I replied that my mother passed away when she was only thirty-six years old. He explained that daughters often have their menopause pretty much around the same time as their mothers, plus or minus a year.

When I returned to the monastery that day, I experienced a deep sadness. All my life I'd never had an urgent desire to have children, but suddenly when I learned that I could be going through early menopause, something in me revolted and resisted the idea. It was as though I no longer had a choice whether or not to have children.

For three days I went through a mental crisis. I felt extremely restless, uneasy, as though I was suffocating, and my mind started to search for a possible person who could have a child with me. It was serious, and at the same time humorous, when I understood the mental state I was in. I learned to breathe with it, relaxing my thoughts and my body and smiling to it. Humor is a great way to deal with stress—here I was a nun and I was scanning for a compatible partner to have a child with as soon as possible. It was completely out of desperation.

As soon as I recognized this, the frantic mental search began to subside. I could smile with myself. To be a nun is my daily choice, and as a nun, I don't have biological children. But the children and teenagers that I work with are my spiritual children. I love them and transmit to them the practice of mindfulness so that they can take good care of themselves. Every time they come to the monastery, they open their arms to embrace me. Sometimes the boys have grown into young men, and when they open their arms to hug me, for a moment I think I can't hug them, because according to our monastic rules of conduct, which we call the "fine manners," monks and nuns don't hug people of the opposite sex. However, if I didn't allow them to hug me, they would be so disappointed and surprised, unnecessarily. So I smile, bow, and hug them. Seeing them as my own children and rejoicing in their growth and progress has helped me to reconcile with the loss of not being able to have my own children. Even though my menstrual cycle normalized after that, I was grateful for the process that I had gone through.

Later, during my first winter at Blue Cliff Monastery in upstate New York, when I was experiencing the worst symptoms of Lyme disease, at one point my period was three weeks late. I saw Dr. Quang, a Vietnamese herbalist in Vermont, who took my pulse and told me I was probably going through early menopause because Lyme disease weakens and changes many processes in one's body.

This time, I didn't experience the same amount of sadness as at Deer Park Monastery, perhaps because I had gone through that process once already. This time I also recognized that I was very sick and tired, and even if I had a chance to bear a child, I wouldn't be healthy enough to take care of my child and to grow with him or her.

Moreover, in moments of both health and sickness, I always cherish my monastic life. Each day I choose to be a nun again and again. It isn't a vow I made on the day I was ordained, but one I choose day after day. So I could accept early menopause more easily this time.

Dr. Quang also told me that it's very important to try to prolong having my periods for as long as I can, because more toxins and bacteria are excreted through menstruation than through urination, defecation, or sweating.

I had studied medicine and I knew that estrogen helps women with their cardiovascular health; women have less risk of cardiac disease than men, but after menopause their risk is the same as for men. I knew that estrogen helps with bone density, and that it's important for skin health and moods, but I had never considered that menstruation could help with the excretion of toxins from a woman's body so effectively. I had always regarded menstruation as something of an inconvenience and a chore, and I couldn't wait for it to finish each time.

The herbal doctor told me to massage my uterus for a week before the menstrual time, during it, and for one week after, and he emphasized, "The more you bleed, the better." This was a new concept for me. One night as I was massaging and sending kind energy to the uterus, I found myself having a conversation with it. I referred to my uterus as my younger sister.

I said, "My dear one, you have been there for me all these years. You have worked diligently so that I may have the strength and beauty of a young woman, but I have never acknowledged what you have done to serve me. Now my body is weak and you are about to go out. I'm not asking you to stay longer if you can't. I just want to let you know that I am very grateful for you."

Tears streamed down. I felt a deep connection with my body, particularly with my uterus. I had been looking for love outside of myself, but in that moment, I realized love had always been there in my body. My body is indeed the most generous, forgiving, and faithful lover there is to me. It was healing to me because I could touch this love and gratitude in myself for my own body, and it helped me not to resist the loss.

When we lose somebody there is great pain from losing that person, but the greater amount of pain comes from our resistance and denial, even guilt and resentment, for that loss. However, when we face the loss with affection and gratitude and we begin anew with it, then this departure is something sweet, soft, and gentle. We can let go and heal much more easily. Again and again through my illness, I learned to be there and reconcile with my own unskillfulness concerning my own body.

MIRROR NEURONS

When you love another person but you lack understanding and love for yourself, then you may see the other person as merely an outside object that you use to enhance your survival and your sense of self in some way. It's like having a source of food that will enhance your chance of survival if it belongs to you.

You may believe that if a person belongs to you, you will feel more secure and complete. However, if you don't know how to listen to yourself, you won't understand that person's aspirations, desires, happiness, and suffering. You'll have no point of reference.

The Buddha is known for his miraculous power of understanding thoroughly the mind of others. The Buddha attained this ability by knowing his own mind thoroughly. He didn't use the sophisticated instruments that we have nowadays in neuroscience, but he used his own mind as a point of reference to study and understand the mind of others. This is possible because the basic working principles of the mind are the same in everyone.

Neuroscience has found that there are mirror neurons in animal brains that enable them to feel what others are feeling. Whether neuroscientists are able to locate this mirror neuron system in humans or not, we know with certainty that we feel what others are feeling, and their feelings affect us greatly. Sometimes you walk into a room and the mere presence of a particular person may suddenly make you feel threatened or defensive.

We are connected to other human beings, feeling what others feel in our own body and mind. However, it's only with self-awareness that we're able to respond empathically and appropriately. When a feeling arises and you simply assume it, then you are its victim. Recognizing another person's emotion and taking care of it in your own body is part of being your own soul mate, knowing yourself, remembering yourself, and mastering your own thoughts, feelings, and perceptions as they arise.

The first step is to call the feeling by its true name, such as anger, sadness, suspicion, desire, etc. With mindful breathing, you can relax your body and mind so that you aren't compelled to react to that feeling or to that person through your thoughts, words, and bodily actions. In this process, you may be able to identify the source of that feeling to see whether it's arising from yourself or from the other person. Self-awareness is also protective, helping us to remain empathetic to others when they're depressed without internalizing their depression within ourselves.

On the other hand, if we're too preoccupied by our own thoughts or strong emotions, then we may not be able to perceive and experience the feelings of the other person. For example, a child is playing at home, and she hears the slamming of doors, heavy footsteps. Her father walks in, and she senses his anger immediately. The child may become frightened or confused. If the father is mindful, he in turn will feel his child's confusion and fear, and he will be able to calm himself down in order to comfort her. However, if too preoccupied with his own frustration and anger from work, he may not even notice the presence of his child, let alone her desperate feelings. Sometimes a parent may even scream or beat a child mercilessly, not registering the physical and psychological trauma that the child is going through.

CHILDHOOD FRIEND

From the sixth to the tenth grade, I had a good friend named Da Thao, which literally means Night Plant in English. We looked somewhat like each other, and people used to call us twins. Da Thao's parents had a flourishing business, whereas my grandmother had only a tiny shop and barely made ends meet while trying to raise my brother and me.

Da Thao was always generous, kind, and protective of me. Being a little bigger than me, she rode me everywhere on the back of her bicycle, to school and after school. She would buy food for both of us from the street vendors, and I never had to feel bad that I didn't have pocket money.

One day, I was wearing a red dress with a low-cut neck, bought by my mother before she disappeared, and as I happened to bend down to pick up something, Da Thao saw that I wasn't wearing a bra. I was already fourteen or fifteen years old, but neither my grandmother nor I ever thought about the need for a bra for me. Da Thao went home and got her brand new bra to give to me. So my first bra didn't come from my mother but from my friend.

When I went to the United States, amongst the few clothes that I'd brought with me, was my friend's bra, which I still keep until this day. Da

Thao later went to France. During all these years, she has always tried to seek me out and keep in touch with me. She missed my ordination at Plum Village Monastery in France, but she came right afterward and visited me a few more times.

After I left Plum Village to go to Deer Park Monastery, Da Thao went to the United States to visit her friends and she also looked me up. She has treated me as her best friend and also as her own sister. Her friendship and kinship has comforted me and protected me since I was a young girl. Perhaps I've experienced much sadness and losses in my life, but I've also been blessed to have friends like her to support me and shape the person I have become.

BEAUTIFUL AS YOU ARE

In college, young men pursued me, but because of my sexual trauma I was always afraid and cautious toward men who were a few years older than me; I considered them to be old men, and I wanted nothing to do with them romantically. I was singularly focused on my studies, because my grandmother wanted me to obtain a higher education.

Then, while I was tutoring chemistry students, I met a young man who was three years younger than me. He kept talking to me and pursuing me, and he became my first boyfriend when I was in my junior year in college. Rob was also a good friend to me, loving and accepting. When I was studying for the MCAT, this young man would come early in the morning to my dorm with three warm bagels in a paper bag. He drove me to the library, and there, he secretly tore these bagels into small pieces so

I could have easy access to them and munch on them discreetly while I was studying. He wished the best for me and nothing for himself. Because I was studying, I wasn't spending time with him. He would leave me alone to study the whole day and come to pick me up afterward.

Back then, I didn't wear much makeup, just some eye shadow and lipstick sometimes; I felt I didn't have time for those things because I was busy studying. I did feel self-conscious when I compared myself to other young ladies who were dressing up beautifully and wearing a lot of makeup.

One day this young man simply said to me, "Huong, you are very beautiful. You don't need to wear makeup at all." Something in the way he said it lifted all my complexes. I no longer felt the need to wear makeup, and if I did, it was just to be funky and fun.

I was thankful to Rob, the first young man I dated, because his positive attitude helped free me from complexes that I might have had about my body. Many teenage girls and young women wear a lot of makeup because they don't appreciate and accept their own look. This is a message of rejection to their own bodies, and it's damaging. Nowadays when I work with young people, I often advise the young men to encourage their female friends and partners to recognize and foster their natural outer and inner beauty. One young friend shared that after she stopped wearing makeup for a few months, her skin became visibly clear, soft, and rosy. She looked at herself in the mirror and a thought arose, "I am so beautiful, my forehead, my eyes, my nose, my mouth..." And she cried.

HUGGING A PROSTITUTE

While I was attending medical school in San Francisco, I often went to a Vietnamese restaurant in a dilapidated neighborhood. There were many drug users and prostitutes walking on the street. One night as we were driving slowly away from the restaurant, I saw a woman walking in the direction of our car. She was just skin and bones, and her short skirt showed her scrawny legs. She was no older than in her thirties, and yet her facial skin was obviously discolored and unhealthy despite the covering of makeup she had on. Her teeth were yellow and unsound, and some were already missing, which made her look even more haggard and elderly. These were the teeth of a cocaine addict; they had become discolored, the gums had also weakened, and the teeth had gotten uprooted prematurely.

I asked my friend to stop the car. I walked toward her, and when I was in front of her, I said, "May I give you a hug?" The woman was speechless. I opened my arms and embraced her scrawny body. Her body stiffened and then after a while, it softened a little more. I didn't know anything about hugging meditation at that time, but there was love in my heart for this woman and for her body. There was no obstacle between her and me. There was no discrimination and no difference between us. I held her in my arms, and I felt her in my body and I felt this oneness with her. All I said to her was, "Please take care of yourself." Then I smiled to her and walked back to the car. She was somebody who wasn't a friend of her body, who didn't know the deep value of her own body, and because of life circumstances, she had to use her body in exchange for drugs, food, and shelter.

Hugging can be a healing meditation practice. Breathe in and out in mindfulness at least three times as you look at the other person. This may be a moment of Noble Silence, when body and mind are fully present, still, and relaxed. Then you embrace each other. There is no need to pat each other's shoulder or to say anything. Simply breathe. Give rise to the awareness that the other person is alive and in your arms. Give rise to love and gratitude. There have been times that my relationship with one of the monastic sisters is strained or hurtful. Words may just stir up more pain. If my sister would allow me, I would simply hold her in my arms and pray silently, "I am sorry. Help me to love you as you are."

LOVE FOR THE CHICKEN

I had been a nun for three years when I went home to visit my brother for the first time. One day while he was away at work, I opened his freezer and saw many meat packages that were about to expire. After looking at those packages for a while, I took out some chicken, thawed, marinated, and cooked it.

I had cooked this dish for my brother many times before I was ordained. When he came home, the meal was ready, with rice, salted chicken and some vegetables. My brother ate happily and quickly, while I just ate my vegetarian food quietly next to him.

I was never a vegetarian before I became a nun, but since I was ordained, I haven't missed eating meat at all, except one time. As I smiled and remembered why I chose not to eat meat, the craving subsided.

When my brother finished his meal, he looked at me and said,

"Sister, I thought as a nun you don't cook meat." I replied, "I don't."

"But you cooked meat for me," he said. And I told him, "When I looked at the meat packages that were about to expire, I thought of you. Every morning you wake up before four o'clock to go to work, and you don't come home until later in the day. You work so hard to have this house, but you never have time to enjoy it. You work so hard to buy everything you have, including the meat, but you don't even have time to cook it and eat it. So out of love for you I cooked this meat. It's also out of love for the chicken that I cooked it, because it was killed for you. But if you don't eat it and you throw it into the garbage, then it's been betrayed twice. These are the reasons I cooked the meat for you."

I also explained to my brother that it was not because I hated meat that I didn't eat it, but it was because of the practice of love for the animals, who also want to live. My brother remained silent. For years after that, every time I came home to see him, I would see only a few meat packages in his freezer.

We use mindful manners and precepts to guide our actions, but on the other hand, there's a teaching that we should not be caught up in precepts and in rituals. As monastic practitioners, we aren't allowed to cook meat. However, I saw the interbeing nature between my brother and the chicken, and I was then able to cook the meat with love for the chicken and also for my brother.

In the teaching of the Buddha, we can realize love at every level. Love is not rigidly formulated, but happens spontaneously. Love is not an effort that we have to make in every moment. On the contrary, mindfulness of love and the insight of interbeing guide our actions, and in turn, our actions take place naturally.

CAT WOMAN

During the skit and performance night at the end of one of our 2010 retreats at Deer Park Monastery, we saw an interesting play. A talented young woman played the role of a little mouse that wanted to become a cat. The mouse became a cat, went through the whole experience of being a cat, and, in the end, it came back to the form of the mouse.

The young woman playing the cat was lithe, joyful, and mischievous, and I was impressed with her talent. Afterward, I said something to her, meaning to praise her, but somehow—perhaps the way I pronounced a certain word unclearly—she misunderstood it. The next day, she came to me and asked me what I had meant. I can't now remember what word she thought I had said to her, but I laughed and said, "No, that wasn't what I meant. I meant to praise you."

That was our only encounter. A few months later, I was informed that this young woman was dying in the hospital. She had admitted herself into the psychiatric ward there, but then one day, she escaped and ran onto the freeway, and a car hit her. She had been in a coma ever since. Her close friend, who had been going to Deer Park Monastery for many years, told me that this young woman had been in a play, and I immediately knew who she was.

We sent compassionate and peaceful energy to her through our chanting and prayers. More than forty young adults from that retreat returned to Deer Park one weekend to practice and support her and each other.

I went with her close friend to the hospital to see her before she was taken off the respirator. At first, her friend and I were not allowed to go into her room, so we stayed in the lounge nearby. Instead of feeling disappointed or frustrated, I began to sing "Beginning Anew with Water." Thay had translated this ancient Buddhist practice into English, and Sister Trung Nghiem had written music to it. I sang:

At the foot of the mountain
there is a stream.
Take the water from the stream and wash yourself
and you will be cured.
You are the cure.

Under the soles of your feet
there is a stream.
Take a step
on the Earth.
Don't you feel the stream?
And you'll be free.
You are free.

In the heart of great beings
there is a stream.

Let it flow.
Let it be the ground
of your being.
And you'll be loved.
You are love.
You are love.
You are love.

Our Teacher often draws a circle to illustrate consciousness as explained by Buddhist psychology. According to this model, our consciousness has two parts. Just as the ocean has a surface level and the deeper part that in some places goes down thousands of feet, consciousness also has an upper level called "mind consciousness" and a lower level called "store consciousness." It has this name because it holds and stores everything about us. It contains all the seeds that have been transmitted by our ancestors.

Mind consciousness can be in different states. When mind consciousness is in a state of mindfulness, we have a chance to see something as it is, as it arises in that moment. We are able to be aware of our body and of the feelings, perceptions, and mental formations that are surfacing on the level of mind consciousness.

Mindfulness is like water coming from the great source of our enlightened nature; it helps us wash away our wrong perceptions and cool our painful feelings and mental formations. In our daily practice, we generate mindfulness, which works most directly at the level of our mind consciousness.

With persistent mindfulness, mind consciousness can be in a state of concentration and insight. We can touch these bright states of mind throughout the day. Without self-awareness, mind consciousness may be left in a state of dispersion. Unfortunately, many of us are in a state of dispersion, forgetfulness, or oblivion most of the day and most of our lives. Mind consciousness can also be in a state of psychosis, such as hallucination and delusion, which can be triggered by extremely high fever, by certain drugs, or by certain brain tumors.

When we sleep or when we're in a coma, mind consciousness may or may not be present in order to be aware of what is going on inside us and around us.

For example, some people leave the television on all night because they can't sleep without it. They aren't aware of what's on the television, yet images and sounds from the television continue to bypass their mind consciousness and enter their store consciousness, triggering disturbing dreamlike states as if the images and sounds were projected from the store consciousness itself. During sleep, mind consciousness may or may not be present to be aware of what is going on, but we continue to receive input, which affects the quality of our sleep. When the television is on day and night, whether or not we're paying attention to it, it becomes the background noise of our consciousness, watering seeds and triggering negative mental states in us.

Caretakers may use the television to entertain and soothe babies and children, but as they're constantly exposed to these flashing images and sounds, their brain development is inevitably affected.

In coma, as in sleep, a person's mind consciousness may or may not be there to know what's going on. He or she may not be able to say anything or to move at all. Yet store consciousness continues to be at work, and consequently, all inputs may still be downloaded into it. Thus, we should maintain a respectful, peaceful, and loving environment for a person in a coma. We can show our care and affection by gently stroking the person's face or massaging his or her hands and feet. We can share with that person our gratitude, the beautiful memories and the things that we feel we need to say.

When we witness the last moment of a person's life, it's unlikely we'll be able to be present for that person if we're uncomfortable with our own death, if we haven't practiced looking at ourselves and our fear, attachment, and desire. In that case, when it's the last moment of our own life, we won't be able to be present either. In their final moments, some people experience hallucinations or delusions, some scream or cry; others slip into oblivion under the influence of morphine. These kinds of endings occur because during our lifetime we aren't tending to our store consciousness, we aren't taking care of the input and the output, and so in the final moments of our life, when all barriers are lifted and socialization, culture, and self-inhibition are all removed, then past memories and unfinished business surge up from store consciousness and take over. The implosion can be devastating.

When I was allowed to go into the room to see the young woman in a coma, I sat quietly next to her bed. Her best friend, who had been in the room with her all along, was playing some music that they used to listen to together. I simply followed my own breathing while observing her breathing pattern. She had been taken off the respirator, and she continued to breathe on her own for almost three-and-a-half hours.

The breathing pattern of a dying person is characteristic: all respiratory muscles are used, and the airway makes loud, drawn out noises, "heh-eh-eh-eh," then, "haw-aw-aw-aw." It's as if the entire body is investing its last drops of energy into breathing. I anchored myself in my own breath, calming my feelings and perceptions, so that I could be fully present with her in these monumental moments of her life.

Suddenly, her breathing quickened and her hands turned ash white. Her friend said, "Sister! Look at her hands! What's happening?" I gently whispered, "The time is coming." I asked her best friend to turn off the music. It was important in that moment that the environment was quiet and peaceful so that her consciousness could remain calm. In such a moment, people who are present in the room shouldn't talk, cry, chatter, or be distracted by anything else.

Everything was calm and still and present. On the monitor, the cardiac waves started to become disturbed and distorted. The oxygen levels started to plummet to the eighties, seventies, sixties. . . . Two of her friends held her hands. I sat on her bed, placing one hand on her chest and the other on her face. I guided her with words from the chant of "Beginning Anew with Water":

And you are cured, and you are cured, and you are the cure.
And you are free, and you are free, and you are free.

Let go off your sadness, my dear.

Let down your burdens, my dear.

Let them go.

Put them down.

It's okay. It's okay.

And you are free, and you are free, and you are free.

And you are loved, and you are love, and you are love.

I sang this song to her in a deep voice, again and again. Then I did a guided meditation, saying that this water could purify all of her sadness and confusion. With her heart pure and light and open, she could now allow her body to rest. I told her how much she was loved, and how much joy she had brought to the world. Even though she was at Deer Park only that one time doing the skit, she had brought so much laughter to us, and all of us were so impressed by her talent, her joy, and her deep insight.

I talked to her gently, massaging her hands and touching her face. Her eyes and her mouth were wide open. She wasn't aware of anything that was going on at the level of mind consciousness, but I continued to speak to her because her store consciousness could still receive and register input.

I walked her through, while I was keenly aware of my own breath and of her breath. "It's okay, my dear. Let go of your sadness. Let down your burdens."

Her breathing pattern became even deeper and more laborious. Her blood pressure began to drop rapidly. Her cardiac waves were changing quickly. She was going to die at any moment. I continued to tell her,

"There is peace in you. Touch that peace in you. Touch that calm in you. Touch that spaciousness in you. You are free. You are free. There is no more sadness. There is nothing to hold onto. You are a beautiful child of Mother Earth, and you are coming back to Mother Earth." I then sang to her:

> I entrust myself
> I entrust myself
> to the Earth
> to the Earth
> and she entrusts herself to me.

Then I changed the words to, "I entrust myself to the Buddha . . ." "I entrust myself to the Dharma . . ." and, "I entrust myself to the Sangha . . ." Then, "I entrust myself to Peace . . ." "I entrust myself to Love . . ."

She struggled, because the cause of her demise was violent, because her young life was full of sadness and turbulence. In her dying moments, the struggle continued. She had stopped breathing and we thought that was the end, but then she started breathing and gasping for air again, and she did that five, six, seven, eight, nine times.

She stopped for a long pause, and then she started again. Even when the heart line went flat, the oxygen levels completely dropped, and the machine beeped frantically, there was still breathing, and there was still gasping for air!

Her eyes were wide open like fish eyes, from the severe brain damage,

peace. We will continue you. We will live beautifully and mindfully for

but I believed that it was also the unresolved conflicts and unfinished business of her life that caused this constant struggling and gasping even into her death. I turned toward the top of her bed and put my hand on her forehead, stroking her forehead and stroking down her eyes. I whispered, "It's okay. Let go, my love. Let go, and you are at peace, and you are peace. We will continue you. We will live beautifully and mindfully for you. We will help you heal your pain—the pain that you haven't been able to heal."

Then I evoked the name of the Bodhisattva of Deep Listening and Great Compassion, Avalokiteshvara, as I continued to stroke her face and close her eyes. It was to help her to pass on peacefully and let go, because at that moment, it was still not too late for her to let go and touch peace.

Her mouth was still wide open. I stroked her upper lip and brought up her lower jaw so that it could close a little more. It was also out of kindness for her parents and loved ones. They would have to view her, and if her eyes and mouth were wide open like that, it would cause them further sadness and pain.

Her forehead began to turn deathly pale too, and the sweat wasn't like when you're hot and you sweat; the sweat oozing from her forehead and her face was sticky and clammy. Bear with that. It is your own death. You are there to witness not only another person's death but also your own. Learn to be present for it.

This was all part of the dying process, but probably it was also because there were certain unresolved things in her life that she could not let go of. So I gently said to her, "Let it go. Let it go. My dear, let it go." I caressed her face ever so gently, and finally she passed away.

Finally, she exhaled three times, "haah!" then "haah!" then "haah!" All was quiet. Her face looked peaceful and serene. Her eyes were closed. There was no distortion or contortion of her face or of her body.

As we learn about our consciousness, we begin to take better care of our body and mind. We become aware of the input and output, of our retributions, and we look deeply into our arising feelings, perceptions, and mental formations. This is not a luxury. This is not about "when I have time, I will meditate" or "when I am older, I will tend to my mind." This is a matter of life and death—right in this very moment, and in every moment of our life.

If we learn to be our own soul mate, our own friend and kin, present for our body, feelings, perceptions, mental formations, and consciousness, then we're present for life, and we can live a beautiful life, regardless of our profession or status. You can be a doctor and then become a nun, and it isn't a wasted effort. You can be a janitor or you can be an engineer or you can be whatever you are—these are all only skillful means for you to live this life, to discover this life in you and around you.

Many young people don't know what direction they're going to follow, and even when we're older, many of us still don't know. We're on a horse, racing through life. "Where are you going?" "I don't know! Ask the horse!" The horse can be a career, fame, success, whatever we think it should be, or whatever our parents and society might think it should be; these are all only skillful means to discover life, they are not life itself. When you are at the moment of death, whether of somebody else or of yourself, all those things fall apart. They mean nothing!

All that matters at that moment is how we've lived our life; how we've cared for our five aggregates of body, feelings, perceptions, mental formations, and consciousness, and how we've cared for other people's five aggregates. Only these things determine the quality of our life, and they will determine the quality of our death and of our continuation.

If someone witnesses a violent or frightful death, that person may then be fearful of death. On the other hand, if that person witnesses someone being able to be there for her own peaceful, beautiful death, that person will neither fear life nor death. To be fully present is what matters.

As a community of practitioners, we support each other and help make our lives more beautiful and meaningful in every moment. With mindfulness in your daily life, you can see when the mind is like a horse that's out of control and is carrying you away. You can ask yourself, and others, the question, "Where are you going?" A ten-year-old child at a retreat wisely responded to this question, "When you ask, it will stop." This is transformation at the base.

Chapter Three

JOY

The sky is deeper blue today, because I have awareness.
The trees are more alive today, as I breathe in their greenness.
The birds are soaring higher, with my eyes following their path.
The children's laughter is brighter, as my own lips are blooming.
And you, you are closer to me than ever, because I know myself more.

Another element of true love is "mudita," or joy. If you love someone, and you often make that person worried, anxious, angry, insecure, or sad, then it isn't true love. In true love, the lover, the beloved, and the love are imbued with joy and happiness.

In the Buddhist context, there's a fine distinction between joy and happiness. Joy is a feeling that may still contain some excitement and anticipation, whereas happiness is a feeling that has reached a state of coolness and calm.

For example, if a person traversing the desert is deeply thirsty, and suddenly in the distance sees some palm trees and the possibility of an oasis, there's hope for water and a feeling of joy arises in anticipation of being able to drink. Such a feeling of joy still contains some excitement and restless movements of body and mind.

But once the person gets to the oasis, kneels down, scoops the water, and drinks it slowly, the water cools the entire body, and the person feels completely at ease and restful. Thirst has been quenched. There's no more seeking. That is a moment of happiness.

Similarly, you can feel joy in the anticipation of meeting or seeing someone. Once you are established in deep connection with that person, you can simply be in the same space, sitting next to each other, without the need to say or to do anything. This complete ease and comfort with oneself and with another person is a moment of deep happiness.

Joy and happiness are essential elements of the Buddhist path. In the Four Noble Truths, the first two Noble Truths are about recognizing the presence of suffering and understanding its causes and conditions. This understanding brings us to the path leading to true joy and happiness, the fourth Noble Truth. Suffering here is seen as noble, because it can help us gain profound understanding of the working of our mind, thus transforming our deeply ingrained habit energies and wrong perceptions.

The prognosis made by the Buddha in the third Noble Truth is that suffering can be completely cured, and this complete cessation of suffering is the full manifestation of joy and happiness.

If we're lost in a dark forest and we see a light in the distance, we immediately feel much hope and joy. Similarly, the awareness that there is a path of practice that can transform and heal our suffering immediately imbues us with the joy and the energy necessary to go forward and to apply that practice in our daily life, even though we may still have challenges and difficulties ahead.

In addition to the Four Noble Truths, many other important teachings of the Buddha also emphasize the importance of joy on the path of practice, and joy is considered to be one of the Seven Factors of Awakening.

There is a Vietnamese proverb, "Waiting for the fig to fall into your mouth." There's a lazy man lying underneath a fig tree; all the figs are ripe, but he's too lazy to pick them, so he lies there with his mouth open waiting for the figs to fall. Conditions of joy and happiness are always available like the ripened figs, but we have to pluck them, enjoy them, and share with others.

PRACTICES FOR GENERATING JOY AND HAPPINESS

Thay often says that true practitioners are able to generate a moment of joy and happiness any time they want, and there are concrete ways that the Buddha has proposed, in particular the practices of Letting Go, Mindfulness, Concentration, and Insight.

Letting Go

Squirrel and the Ten-Foot Pole

In the spring of 2014, Sister Bamboo decided to buy seeds to feed the yellow-breasted finch. We have a balcony in front of our nunnery, so

Sister Bamboo tied a wooden stick to a corner of the balcony and hung the bag of seeds off the end of the stick. Nothing happened the first two weeks. Then lo and behold, the yellow-breasted finches arrived. They sang beautiful childlike, high-pitched songs, and they pecked daintily at the bag of seeds. Another week or so went by. Some squirrels began to gather on the deck. They climbed the wooden stick and tore the bag, so all the seeds were scattered on the ground. Sister Bamboo stitched up the bag, but then the squirrels tore it open again. She asked for my advice. I told her that a metal rod might be too slippery for the squirrels to climb. She found a thin metal rod that bent at the end like an L, and a plastic tube that we usually use for "stick exercises"— ten tai chi movements we do while holding a long stick, usually bamboo, in both hands. She stuck the metal rod into the plastic tube, which she then tied to the corner of the balcony. Now we had the bag of seeds hanging off a ten-foot pole, dangling in midair. Just to make sure that it would deter the squirrels, Sister Bamboo oiled the plastic tube with Vaseline. Imagine the squirrels trying to get to the bag of seeds! They would jump up as high as they could, only to slide back down because of the Vaseline. Some even tried to bypass the plastic tube! The sisters had great fun watching the squirrels doing acrobatics.

One day Sister Sun Rise and I were sitting on the porch and enjoying the scene. One squirrel was content to eat the seeds from the balcony floor, but another squirrel was determined to climb up the pole. After each attempt, the squirrel would pause to look at the bag of seeds. It was so high up in the air that the squirrel had to tilt its head all the way back at such a sharp angle that it could have fallen on its back any time. I spoke for that squirrel, "Dear bag of seeds, you are so great. I want you so badly. I would do anything for you, even break my back, my neck, literally." Sister Sun Rise said, "The seeds on the ground and the seeds in the bag are the same." I replied, "Oh no! If the seeds on the ground are that good, the seeds in the bag must be ten times better!" So back and forth, Sister Sun Rise and I were singing love songs about lovers yearning for each other and talking in squirrel-like voices. By the end, we agreed that probably the squirrels were thinking, "The nuns are evil!"

Amidst all that joy and fun, I thought to myself, "How am I different from that squirrel? What is the great bag that I'm pursuing?" What is that great bag for you? Is it a diploma or another degree? Is it some situation? Is it someone? Do you know how to enjoy the wonderful seeds that are already available to you?

The first principle of cultivating joy and transforming suffering is that joy and happiness are born from letting go (*ly sinh hy lac*). This may seem counterintuitive, especially in our modern society, where consumption is believed to be the answer to everything.

Let us imagine a person feeling confined and suffocated in a noisy and crowded city, who one afternoon decides to drive to the countryside. As soon as he leaves the city and enters the countryside, the sight of bright flowers in the meadow, the open space, and the crisp air shower him with pleasant sensations. He can breathe more easily, and he immediately feels a sense of well-being and ease at having left the city behind.

Similarly, in letting go, we release the many, many things that are crowding our outer and inner space. We simplify our possessions, such as clothing, decorations, and electronic gadgets. We may have a busy schedule, but when we pause to look into our activities and prioritize them, we may recognize that certain meetings, parties, and engagements only distract us and take away our time. We can let go of them to simplify our life and to have more time, space, and energy for ourselves and for our loved ones.

One monastic brother shared that when his sister was happy she'd gotten a promotion at work, he was quietly wishing that she'd gotten a demotion instead, because with a promotion, she would have to work harder to prove herself worthy of that position. She'd be taking on many more responsibilities and would thus have less time for herself and her family.

Knowing that you have enough is a practice that brings much joy and happiness. When we have time to stop and look deeply, we can experience the joy that is already there.

Releasing Ideas and Views

It used to be important to me to be right and to prove my point. Since I've become a practitioner, I see that right or wrong are just relative; they also have the interbeing nature. Something may seem so right in this moment, but at another time it's no longer that important. When you learn to look at it from different angles you realize why people think or do things differently from you. You see yourself in that situation, too. At this moment you say, "I'm this kind of person and I only do this." Yet a few months or years later you may do the exact opposite. Previously you'd said, "I'm not the type of person who would do that," and yet you do it now because the time is different, the situation is different, and you are different. Right and wrong are relative, and they inter-are. We learn to be more tolerant and open to possibilities.

Letting go of views is a deep kindness that we can practice with our beloved. In true love, we should strive for harmony, rather than try to prove that we're right and the other person is wrong. Harmony is first of all for the sake of our own body and mind. When we fight with each other we cause physical stress to our body, and our immune system becomes weaker. These arguments continue in our minds even when we're apart from each other, so that day and night our body and mind are burdened by stress and pain. When we strive to cultivate harmony, we reconcile and accept the Middle Way.

Relaxing our views with our smile and our mindful in-breath and out-breath can enhance the quality of our being and help save our lives.

Setting Someone Free

Patrick loved me with utmost acceptance and respect. I too loved him dearly, but I would turn away from him and curl up with my own sadness and pain. At first, I blamed him because I felt that he didn't understand me and what I'd gone through in my life. He always tried to listen, but I felt that he couldn't understand me because he came from such a stable and privileged background.

Then slowly I realized that I didn't even understand myself and that I didn't know how to take care of myself. Therefore, I couldn't make him truly happy. When I told him that we shouldn't be together, it saddened him. In the end, he told me, "Huong, all I want is for you to be happy." He helped me to move out of the house. It was a sad day. We moved things out, and then he drove me to the new place and parked the car in front of it. We both sat in the car and cried. We parted not because we didn't love each other, but because I knew I couldn't bring him long-lasting happiness.

I remember one day I came to his clinic—the door to his office was slightly open and I saw him standing by his desk with a recorder, dictating a report about the patient he had just seen. He was wearing his long white physician's robe and he looked handsome and dignified. He symbolized everything I had dreamed of all my life. Here I was, a child without parents, from a poor family, with an abusive history; all I'd ever wanted was to find somebody I loved, who loved me too, so we could have a stable, happy home together. In this way, I would compensate for everything that I had lost or never had. He symbolized all that. This man was so faithful and loving toward me, and I walked away from him. So I stood there, looking at him through the slit of the door and crying for myself and for my broken dream.

When you don't know how to love yourself and take care of your own suffering, then even if you are fortunate enough to find someone who loves you sincerely, you still walk away. You still step all over the person and what he or she offers to you.

Now, as a monastic practitioner, I learn to befriend myself, sitting quietly, walking peacefully, and listening attentively to myself throughout the day. Every moment is a moment to be with my body, with my feelings, and with my perceptions, to remember, to know, and to understand myself better, so that I can better master these feelings, perceptions, and habit energies. Love flows forth much more naturally; it isn't so much of an effort to love or to endure someone.

When you know how to be with yourself, you will know how to be with another person and share joy and love together.

Letting go may also mean setting someone free, someone you may have clung to in order to be happy, but in actuality, it was a relationship that has only brought much suffering to both of you. The relationship doesn't generate joy or peace, but you're afraid that if you let each other go, then you may not have anything left, and you wouldn't know what to do with yourself. There are couples who stay together because of habit energy and because they're afraid of being alone. To be able to support each other's path and transformation may sometimes mean letting go of our grasping and attachment to the other person. Deep joy and happiness may arise from this courageous act.

Breathing Exercise: Letting Go

Breathing in, I am aware that I am breathing in.
Breathing out, I am aware that I am breathing out.

Breathing in, I follow my in-breath all the way through.
Breathing out, I follow my out-breath all the way through.

We train ourselves to be aware of the in-breath as it is coming in. Then we let go of it, as the out-breath takes place.

In order to follow one breath all the way through, the mind must be able to focus on the breath and release all thoughts and feelings that may be arising during the duration of this one breath. Those of us who practice mindfulness of breathing know this is not a simple task!

Mindfulness

Recently, in a question and answer session, someone asked: When we practice meditation, besides becoming more positive and peaceful, do we actually see anything else? Do we actually hear anything else?

In psychiatry, if you hear something that others don't hear, that's called auditory hallucination. If you see something that others don't see, that's called visual hallucination.

In our mindfulness practice, we don't practice to see and hear things that aren't there, that are considered to be paranormal or supernormal phenomena, or some kind of virtual reality.

We don't strive for those things because they actually just come from the mind itself, when it's overstimulated. The neurons in the brain can be overstimulated so they secrete excess neurotransmitters, which can cause us to see and hear things that aren't actually present.

We don't practice in order to have these states of mind. We practice to see things as they are, to hear things as they are, and that is called "suchness." Suchness means: "As it is."

Often, when we look at something, we don't actually see it as it is.

For example, if you look at a flower arrangement, what do you see? Immediately you see a category, "flower," or "tulips." You don't see this phenomenon or this being as it is.

Categories have already been written down and programmed in our brain: these are flowers, these are leaves, these are the branches, this is my wife, this is my child, this is my partner, etc. Scientists call these "invariant categories." They are invariant because they are fixed in our mind, and we only see those categories and not the actual phenomena themselves.

However, in our mindfulness practice, we learn to still and quiet our mind, so that when we open our eyes, we just see that phenomenon as it exists in that very moment. It isn't seen and categorized through the lens of the past, so that we think, "I've seen it before" or "I've known it before." Our seeing isn't based on what we've previously experienced. For example, when you look at a man, your mind might immediately associate him with a past event. He may look like another man who had once been in your life, who brought you joy or pain.

When you hear a sound, do you hear it for what it is, in this very moment? Or do you hear it through the filter of the past as a sound that reminds you of something beautiful, painful, or pleasant?

All of our lives, we're looking and searching, and we continue to do so when we enter spiritual practice. What are we looking for? What are the things we want to see that are extraordinary? What are the things we want to hear that are extraordinary? What are the things we want to experience that are extraordinary? Where do we look for these things?

If you continue to imagine that these things are somewhere "out there," and that you will get there someday, then you may never get there.

The things that we're looking for are already here, right in our body and mind and all around us. We just don't see them and hear them as they are, but we only hear and see invariant categories.

That's why we don't touch the wonders of life. That's why we don't touch the joy and the sacred in everything that is. Coming back to our breathing is something basic and simple, but it enables us to be in touch with life in the here and the now.

We begin to breathe as soon as we're born. If we don't cry, the nurse or doctor will spank us to make us cry and take that first in-breath we need to take on our own. From that moment until now, how many times have we breathed without being aware of it, taking our breath for granted?

Have you ever felt so sick that you could hardly breathe? Your chest is so heavy, your throat is so tight and you are gasping for air. Have you ever gone through that? In that moment what could be more extraordinary than to be able to breathe normally? All you wish is to be able to breathe on your own. When something is there, and we take it for granted, or we aren't mindful of it, then it's ordinary and mundane. But when we're mindful and grateful, we find joy in that very same thing, and we see it as sacred.

Can you see that? It's the same phenomenon in both cases. When you aren't there, it means nothing, but when you're there wholeheartedly, your mind is quiet and calm, then you experience what is, just as it is; that's all the joy and sacredness that you can ever find.

Mindfulness and gratitude are all that's required. But many people don't want to go through that. They want something quicker and more extraordinary. Nevertheless, in my experience, it's in the daily, ordinary, and mundane things, it's in living moment to moment, breath to breath that we touch joy and the sacred and we see meaning in life.

STILL HERE

I have written my best poem
in my sleep.
I knew it, because I told myself so.

I have written my best song
in my dream.
I even tried to memorize it
but I forgot the words the moment I woke up.

So I do my best
to live my ordinary life.
Through each breath
however comfortable or shortened it may be—
In this body
although pain and weariness can be relentless at times—
In each interaction
knowing it is the last—
Holding and gently embracing the tears and the laughter.

And I have touched the most
exquisite love
in these wakeful moments.

—Blue Cliff Monastery, Winter 2013

Breath Is Mind Itself

At a retreat for the Order of Interbeing members, who are long-term practitioners in the Plum Village tradition, a woman asked how to maintain stability when one has much suffering. In response, I asked how many people in the audience actually practiced stopping when they heard the phone ringing in their daily life. Less than five people raised their hands. I told our friends that our Teacher has talked about the practice of stopping with the sound of the bell and of the phone at every orientation session and in many Dharma talks over the last thirty years. Yet few of us actually practice it when we aren't at the monastery.

Perhaps this is because we're afraid that other people may look at us strangely for stopping with the sound of the phone ring. It also may be because we think what we're doing is too important to stop at the moment when the phone is ringing.

It's also our habit energy of running and grasping that doesn't allow us to stop for even two or three breaths. By allowing these habit energies to dictate our thoughts, actions, and speech, we feed and perpetuate our own suffering. We may complain that we suffer, but in fact, many of us are addicted to it. We guard it with all our might by our habitual ways of living and thinking.

As a spiritual practitioner, if you don't cultivate awareness of breathing, you can't go far in the understanding of your mind. In Chinese, the character 息 for "breath" is telling. In this character for "breath," the 自 means "from" or "itself," and the 心 means "the mind." It signifies: "The breath is from the mind. The breath is the mind itself." You can understand this physiologically. When you are angry, you breathe rapidly, and your breath is shallow. When you're sad, you sigh, and your breath is drawn out and laborious. Each mental state such as sadness, despair, anger, or excitement is manifested through the breath. Indeed, it's from the mind that the breath manifests, and it's the mind itself that the breath is manifesting. The mind itself is abstract and elusive. We can't use a finger to point to the mind. The breath, on the other hand, is observable. We can see our breath on cold days. We can taste the breath, smell the breath (hopefully not too much), hear the breath, and touch the breath. Through the five sense organs, we can be in contact with the breath. Undoubtedly, it's comforting and beneficial to befriend our mind through our breath.

In our breathing exercises, at first we practice to be aware of our natural in-breath and out-breath. This is a cultivation of mindfulness—awareness of something as it is in the moment. Then, we practice following each in-breath from the beginning to the end, and following each out-breath from the beginning to the end. This progression is necessary because each breath takes about three to five seconds, and it takes only a split second to identify an in-breath or an out-breath; thus, the mind still has the rest of the time to think and to wander off! This second exercise trains us to string the beads of mindfulness into a beautiful necklace of concentration. Following the breath all the way through is a great challenge, even for just a few breaths! Recognizing our restless mind is to have more love and empathy for ourselves and to cultivate concentration more diligently in our daily lives.

Stopping with the Bell

In our tradition, every time we hear a sound of the bell, the ring of the telephone or the chime of the clock, we stop speaking and doing things in order to return to our breathing. This practice of stopping with the sound of the bell trains us to be aware of and to let go of thoughts and feelings that arise throughout the day. If we can't do this with these small daily sounds, then we'll have no chance to master and release a strong emotion when it surges as a gigantic wave. We're swept away by the strong emotion so completely that we identify ourselves with it. We defend it, and our words and bodily actions may destroy everything that we've worked for in our relationships.

The capacity to stop the chattering mind so it can dwell fully in the present moment determines our capacity to let go of suffering and to touch joy and happiness.

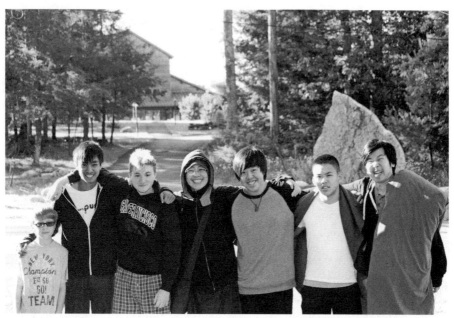

SISTER D AND TEENS

Home Is Here and Now

A group of Korean friends came to visit Blue Cliff Monastery for a few hours. They received a short orientation, went on walking meditation with the Sangha, and had a session of deep relaxation. Their last activity was a session of questions and answers, and I had been asked to be a part of the panel.

Before I left my room to attend this activity, I had a bout of explosive diarrhea. This had been going on for a year, even after I had stopped taking the antibiotics for Lyme disease. It was so painful that I sat still on the toilet for a long while, breathing and relaxing my body. I thanked my body, "Thank you, my dear, for being able to endure this pain. Thank you."

This gratitude enabled me to endure the physical pain without feeling sad or inconvenienced or afraid. When I tried to stand up, the spasm in the anal muscles was so painful that I had to stand still and massage it for a while before I could wash my hands and put on my robe.

On my way to the meditation hall, I took just one step with each breath because there was still spasm and pain. As I was breathing and walking mindfully, I was aware of the soft sunlight and of the flowers growing along the sidewalk. A woman was walking quickly in front of me. It was a beautiful day.

By the time I entered the meditation hall and bowed toward the altar, everyone else was already seated in a circle. I walked slowly around the circle, to an empty cushion my sister had reserved for me by her side and by the bell.

I stood behind the cushion, bowed, and silently recited the gatha,

> Sitting here
> is like sitting under a Bodhi tree.
> My body is mindfulness itself,
> free from all distraction.

Then I sat down and adjusted myself so that my body posture could be as upright and relaxed as possible. Without looking at anyone, I kept my gaze downward and stayed with my breathing, a soft half-smile on my lips.

My sisters had already started the session, so I stayed completely quiet so as not to disturb the people due to my late arrival. After a couple of questions, an older Korean gentleman raised his hand and asked permission to address his question to me. He said in English, "Dear sister, I feel in your energy there is a lot of peace, and you are so beautiful that you could be a model. Have you had any realizations? I mean, if you have attained some realizations, would you share with us?"

Some people were chuckling as his question was translated into Korean.

I smiled and all I could think was that I'd just had a severe bout of diarrhea. I was sure I looked extremely pale. Certainly, I wasn't in the best state to consider myself as looking beautiful.

My response was, "All my life I didn't feel that I belonged anywhere. I didn't belong even in my home with my mother and my relatives. I didn't even feel that I belonged in my own homeland, Vietnam. I suffered from the complex of inferiority because I was an Amerasian and looked different from other children, because I didn't have parents, and because I came from a family poorer than those of my friends.

"There were many reasons that prevented me from feeling that I was at home, that I could be accepted in my own home or in my own country.

"When I came to the US, in the eyes of many Americans I looked exotic and different. Even though I tried hard to fit into the American culture, I knew that I could never be completely American because my outward appearance immediately betrayed me.

"When I became a nun, I began to notice that I had many recurrent dreams. The dreams would take different forms but they all had the same theme. I would be somewhere and suddenly I realized I was far away from home and needed to go back home.

"Usually I would see myself in Vietnam, and then I would panic because the plane was taking off soon and I couldn't find my ticket, or I didn't have a ride to the airport.

"Another scenario would be that I was lost somewhere and I didn't know how to find my way back. For years, this had been a recurrent dream.

"After I became a monastic, I continued to have these dreams, but my thinking and reactions in them began to change slowly. When I found that I was lost somewhere in one dream, I said to myself, 'It's okay. If I keep going straight on this road, it will lead me home.' There was a sense of direction and it gave me confidence and ease.

"In another dream, I was trying to keep up with some brothers and sisters in front of me, while we were on our way to a place that had offered us food. People were talking loudly and moving about everywhere, and I was losing sight of my brothers and sisters. I felt lost and became frantic. Suddenly I said to myself, 'It's really not necessary that I have to get there. I don't need to eat that food.' At that moment my pursuit was released and everything slowed down. My whole body felt relaxed and at ease. The throng of people vanished. The space all around me and inside of me became quiet.

"In a recent dream, I was lost in a gigantic store, but I knew that my mother was waiting for me somewhere, that she hadn't just left me alone there. All I needed to do was get back to the front door of the store to find her.

"The fear and pain of the wounded child in me surfaced in my dreams in that way throughout my adult life. Before I embarked on my spiritual journey, I didn't know how to cultivate mindfulness and healing during the daytime, so when those fears and wounds manifested at night, the child in me would experience the trauma of the past all over again. When I woke up, I would again feel the fear, the anxiety, and the sorrow.

"Now that I've been practicing in my daily life, the energy of mindfulness penetrates my sleep, and in my sleep I'm no longer a blind victim. I see the situation more clearly. I respond to it differently and I find a way out. This is a deep transformation that all of us can obtain as practitioners. It is known as 'transformation at the base' in Buddhist psychology.

"In my practice, I've learned that my home isn't in a physical structure, in a roof over my head, or in a particular place in space and time, but home is in the present moment, in the here and the now. Wherever I go, I practice touching home in my steps and in my breath. I practice touching home in Mother Earth, and this practice helps me to dwell more deeply in the present moment and to heal the fear of abandonment, the anxiety about being lost, and the confusion and chaos that I experienced in my childhood. These daily practices have helped heal me in my waking moments, and they have helped transform my perceptions and reactions in my dreams. So if I have attained any sort of realization, I guess it's the realization that home is here and now."

Smile of Nonfear

Another Korean man asked about the meaning of our smiles because he had noticed the half-smiles on the faces of the monastic sisters. Many other people have asked me, "Sister D, are you very happy? You must be very happy because you smile all the time."

I reply that I am indeed happy some of the time, but most of the time I'm simply smiling with myself and with my own thoughts. My thoughts can be joyful and positive, but they can also be ridiculous, startling, and perverse. Instead of reprimanding myself or denying those negative kinds of thoughts, I learn to smile to them; this is the practice of nonfear.

In our practice, we learn not to be afraid of anything, and foremost the things that are coming from inside of us. We may wish ourselves to be wholesome and perfect, but we have to be realistic and see that we're neither entirely wholesome nor perfect. Anything that arises in us— wholesome and perfect, or not—is a part of us, a part of our habituated self. We need only to smile to that thought of jealousy, anger, sadness, desire, or fear and it will subside and lose its strength over time.

As we cultivate this smile of nonfear, we will be able to accept the past and welcome whatever conditions may arise in the present moment or in the future.

When Zen masters die, how is their death different from others? When we are true practitioners and can smile to whatever happens in our daily life, then when the moment of death arrives, we'll be able to have a smile of nonfear because we'll be able to release this body without grasping or regret. In that moment, we can simply follow our breathing until the last out-breath. We leave this world with a smile and continue on in other forms. The question is whether or not we have enough time and true love for ourselves to cultivate this smile of nonfear in our daily life.

When doing sitting meditation, I have observed that many people look tense and their faces may become distorted. Some frown, or purse their lips, or have harsh lines on their forehead or around the mouth. Thay has written a calligraphy: "Breathe and Smile." It's important to be aware of our facial muscles and to relax them with a half-smile, as this helps to relax the whole body as well as the feelings, perceptions, and thoughts that may arise during sitting meditation.

It is important to anchor oneself in the awareness of our breathing and bodily posture, while we maintain a smile to relax all of the physical and mental aspects of ourselves.

In our daily life we can definitely learn to smile more often. Usually, people only smile when they are happy or when they have to perform a social smile. That isn't necessarily the only function of the smile. We can learn to smile even when tears are streaming down our face. We can learn to smile when anger is rising in us or when a harsh thought or feeling is brewing in us. If we remember to breathe and smile, that thought and feeling will lose its momentum and subside quickly. The half-smile also helps us not to take the situation too seriously and especially not to get lost in our views and perceptions, but rather to have more equanimity and clarity to see the situation as it is and to handle it effectively. A smile of equanimity already brings much joy and happiness.

Concentration

Breathing in, I follow my in-breath all the way through.
Breathing out, I follow my out-breath all the way through.

Mindfulness can exist as an instant of awareness, but concentration means that the energy of mindfulness is maintained without interruption over a period of time, just as scattered rays of sunlight can converge into one spot under a magnifying glass and burn a piece of paper.

Similarly, as children, we used to take a piece of plastic wrap and rub it on our pants so that it heated up with concentrated static electricity. Then we held it over little torn pieces of paper, and they danced and jumped and stuck to the plastic as though it were a magnet.

Many of us can sit at the computer or work in the garden for long hours, but this type of concentration is directed onto an object outside of ourselves. In this modern age, the Internet, electronic gadgets, and quick means of communication bombard us with ceaseless information. We're drawn outward and away from our own self-awareness, and many people suffer from attention deficit hyperactivity disorder (ADHD) at some level.

Learning to return to our breathing and anchoring our mind in our breath and body can help us dwell more deeply in the present moment so that peace, joy, and happiness can be touched and sustained.

In one session of questions and answers, a gentleman asked if it's possible to go on a wrong path when we concentrate on our breathing and forget everything else. In response to his concern, I recounted a story. Recently, two of my sisters were at the doctor's office when a woman asked them, "Can you monastic nuns get married? Do you have children?" The woman was appalled to find out that monastics don't get married or have children, saying, "What would happen to the human race if everyone were to do that?"

My young sister replied, "Please don't worry. People like us are very rare."

So I told the gentleman not to worry that he may forget everything if he is too concentrated on his breathing. If you ever try to follow your breath all the way through, you will discover that it isn't at all easy. I asked everyone in the audience to follow their breathing with the sound of the bell and see how many breaths they could stay with. After the exercise, people said that they could only follow two, three, or four breaths at the most before a thought arose and distracted them.

When the energy of mindfulness is concentrated on one particular object and maintained over a period of time, this energy can help us sustain our peace and happiness.

For example, when you see somebody you have been apart from for a while, you hug and kiss each other joyously and say, "How are you? I'm so happy to see you!" But soon after that, if you go back to your worries, projects, and plans, then even though the person might still be in the room with you, the joy and happiness are already gone.

On the other hand, if you're able to concentrate and stay mindful of the fact that your beloved is right there with you and how wonderful and rare it is that you have a chance to be together, then you'll put aside all your mental chattering and worries so you can be truly present with this person, enjoy this moment, and make it last.

It's like eating a cookie. If you eat it all at once, it's gone. However, if you take time to concentrate and look at the cookie, smell it, take a small bite, enjoy the taste and sensation in your mouth, and then look at it as a child would look at the sky or smile at a butterfly, before you slowly take another bite, you can truly appreciate it and retain a lasting impression of it.

The energy of concentration also helps us to stay with the commitments we've made with our loved ones, investing our energy, time, and effort in them and not getting distracted by the novelty and excitement of other things. To love someone is to be truly present for that person.

Insight

After the Vietnam War, many Vietnamese people tried to escape the country and they were known as boatpeople. There's a story of one boat that was stopped by pirates who took everything and left the people out on the sea to die. Luckily, a ship saw the boatpeople and pulled them to a safe place. When they reached shore, one woman cried out in desperation because the pirates had taken all her jewelry. She had only one carat of gold left, which she had managed to hide in her body, and she didn't know how she was going to live by means of it. A man next to her then began jumping and shouting, "How am I going to survive if all I possess in the world is one pair of shorts?" With only the shorts on his body, this man could still be happy because he recognized that his life was intact.

Even though we may have a lot more than this man, we may be thinking desperate thoughts, even of suicide, because we lack insight about what is important in our lives.

Insight derives from the energy of concentration, and it has the capacity to penetrate through ignorance and shatter layers of afflictions as a concentrated beam of light ignites pieces of paper.

When we're in the dark and we don't know where we are, we can feel frightened and in despair. If suddenly we see a light or hear a sound of someone coming—even though we aren't yet out of the situation—joy and hope nevertheless arise. In the same way, insight, or understanding, of our suffering and its causes can bring deep joy and happiness.

In the darkness of confusion, fear itself is what's most menacing and paralyzing. Once there's understanding, fear is removed, and we have the clarity to see what we need to do and what we need to refrain from doing in order to resolve the difficulty or change the situation.

Invariant Representation

Our animal ancestors lived in the wild and faced constant danger, so they learned to perceive things quickly. If they saw a long coil, they couldn't afford to debate at length whether it was a snake or a rope. They reacted immediately in order to increase their chance of survival.

This capacity for quick reaction is deeply ingrained in us as well. The images, sounds, and experiences of our ancestors were recorded in their memories and transmitted down to us, so that we, too, have their great capacity to recognize and react to danger efficiently.

I had never seen a rattlesnake before or heard its rattle, but when I heard a sudden sound while hiking one day in Arizona, I immediately stopped all movement. Only then did I see a snake on a rock about two feet away from me, facing me and rattling. I had chosen the best course of action purely because of my inherited instincts.

When we perceive something, a flower for example, we've already seen similar flowers through the eyes of our ancestors, or perhaps our mother pointed to a flower and said to us, "Flower. Flower." After a while, whenever we see a flower, we recognize it quickly because it matches the image for "flower" in our memory. This happens quickly, which is good for survival, but we may not register the color, texture, and differences between one flower and the next. We just see a category "flower."

Scientists have referred to this prerecorded image as an "invariant category," because the information is written down and fixed in our brain, which exerts top-down control. The moment the eyes contact the form, the information is identified as "flower." This can also happen with "husband," "wife," "good," "bad," and so forth. Further information isn't processed, and so we don't see the thing as it really is in the present moment.

Neuroscientists have studied this phenomenon. The neocortex of the brain contains information that we've been exposed to during our lifetime (and with certainty, it also contains all the images and information that our parents and ancestors witnessed and experienced by way of their eyes, ears, nose, tongue, body, and mind). The brain relies on these prior expectations and experiences to predict and rationalize the new incoming information from the environment, in order to make conclusions and direct responses in the shortest time possible.

Information about perceived objects is sent through the sensory nerves to the cortex of the brain, which has six layers. Information is received in the bottom, (the fifth and sixth) layers, and moves upward toward the processing (first and second) layers. Simultaneously, the top layers send information back down saying, "I've seen something like this before. It's a . . . snake!" These two signal streams meet somewhere in the middle (third or fourth) layers of the cortex, the two information streams blend, and the perception about the object is made. Thus, we "know" that it's a snake as our cortical top-down processing influences empirical incoming perceptions with its expectational bias. This is discussed by Dr. Daniel Siegel in his book *The Mindful Brain*.

This is fast and efficient but it alters our perception, because identification of the object is made without us having paid very close attention to it. We often operate in this mode. "I know; it's my husband." "I know; it's my daughter." "I know; he's about to ask for money." "I know; walking meditation...."

That is why our perceptions are often limited and incorrect. The Buddha said, "Wherever there is perception, there is deception." Thay said something similar, "At least ninety-nine percent of our perception is incorrect." Therefore, Thay added that we should often ask ourselves, "Are you sure?" And if you are sure, "Check again!"

Perception

I was living in the New Hamlet of Plum Village in my second year as a nun. After the Day of Mindfulness, I went to the plum orchard at the edge of our monastery. A hammock was there, and I liked to rest on it or practice chanting. As soon as I sat down on the hammock, I saw a monk standing right in front of me. He was a guest monk, and I had spoken to him briefly a few times before. Apparently, he had followed me from the sister's hamlet to the plum orchard, but I didn't know it! I was shocked, but I still said hello to him.

He felt awkward, and he said to me, "I just want to give you a letter." He gave me a very thick envelope and hurriedly walked away. After a few silent moments, I opened the envelope and read it. At the time I didn't remember that in our fine manners, when a nun receives a letter from somebody of the opposite sex, she should give it to her elder sister to read first.

So I read the letter, in which he praised me and expressed his admiration and affection for me. There were three pages full of words. I couldn't remember them all, but I still can see vividly the drawing he also did of a young woman with a shaved head, standing sideways and wearing a long robe with a side split that went high above the waist.

It could have been a monastic robe, but it could also have been an ao dai, the Vietnamese traditional long dress. The back flap of the robe was flying in the wind. So even though this young woman clearly had a shaved head, the way the cloth was undulating gave the impression that it was her long hair blowing in the wind.

The young woman in the drawing definitely had a beautiful figure, and what struck me the most was that she had a well-developed bosom. I chuckled to myself and said, "This is definitely not mine, and this is definitely not me!"

This incident taught me the lesson that when we admire or have affection for someone, we may not see that person as he or she truly is. Not only can we misperceive the person's dreams, aspirations, sufferings, and difficulties, but even on the most mundane, physical level, we may create our own version of what he or she looks like. The monk had done this drawing supposedly of me, but by looking at the bosom, I knew it wasn't mine. It was totally imagined.

That evening, I burned the letter by my bedside in front of the altar for my grandmother, my mother, and John. I cried and prayed, "Dear John, losing you is painful, and I never want to love this way again. Please help me to never have to go through this pain again."

Soon after that, I received a second letter from the monk. This time I gave it to my Teacher, because I really didn't want to deal with it. It made things easier that I wasn't attracted to that guest monk. The suffering in me was already overwhelming.

After I gave the letter to Thay, I waited to see what he would teach me about it. Thay would usually teach us directly or through a Dharma talk, so at the next Dharma talk I was tuned-in, attentive. Thay talked about the Buddhist sutra, "Repentance and Taking Refuge for Life"—how to repent one's own past misdeeds and make the aspiration to transform suffering and to help others remove their suffering. I was deeply moved by Thay's teaching.

Then, at the end of the talk, Thay casually said, "The Brothers should know that when you write letters to the Sisters, they often let Thay read your letters." That was all he said, but it was enough to alarm everyone.

Later, Thay intentionally created conditions for this brother and me to talk to each other. During one monastic day at Thay's hermitage, he said, "Brother So-and-So, you can sit down and talk to Sister Dang Nghiem. Sister Dang Nghiem, you should talk to this brother."

I was embarrassed. Everybody was on break, and there I was, sitting under a magnolia tree listening to this monk. He talked about his mother and how he felt abandoned by her when he was young. That experience had wounded him deeply, and he had never felt secure in himself. It was also difficult for him to experience love and to give love to others. I listened to him attentively, and at the end I said to him, "I am not the one you truly love. I am just an object of your perception for now. It could be me, and it could be somebody else. I just hope you'll continue to practice so that you can touch true love for yourself."

This experience taught me that when we have a strong feeling for somebody, we shouldn't quickly jump to the conclusion that it's love. We must take time to reflect on how we experienced love during childhood, what we've learned through past relationships, whether or not we know what love really is, and if we've learned to love ourselves.

There is a song by Jason Mraz, titled "Life Is Wonderful," that goes, "It takes no time to fall in love, but it takes you years to know what love is." This insight can help us come back to ourselves and establish a deeper relationship with ourselves. Only then do we have a chance to truly love another person.

We can also apply this insight in situations where someone is attracted to us. We can evaluate more objectively whether that person can listen to us, understand us, and be our friend by examining whether he or she can do this for himself or herself.

Who Is My Beloved?

In a personal relationship, insight, or understanding of ourselves and of our beloved, will help us to cherish each other and help each other transform habit energies that may be obstacles to our joy and happiness.

You can ask the person you love, silently or directly, "Who are you? Who are you to be with me? Why do you put up with me and go through difficulties with me?"

Not everybody is willing to be with us. After all, most of us often neglect and desert ourselves. If we know we have someone who's there for us through thick and thin, that in itself brings a lot of gratitude and happiness. We learn not to take each other's presence for granted or to think that we can find new joy and happiness in a new relationship.

I once saw on a billboard in San Francisco, "Wherever you go, there you are." Our habit energies and suffering are like stains on an eraser that would smear a new white board. They remain there until we transform them in our own mind. Seeing that the conditions of happiness are already present, we come back to acknowledge and invest further in ourselves and in our relationship.

For various reasons, many people first come to spiritual practice without their partners. With time, their partners become curious about the practice because they see a blossoming freshness, joy, and understanding that for a long time hadn't been in the practicing partner. Then they both come to the monastery and attend retreats. It's always a great joy to see couples and families practicing together.

When we understand reality as it is, we're able to let go of wrong views, misunderstandings, and misperceptions. In letting go of these negative mental formations, we touch a deep well of joy and happiness. Without this joy we can't develop concentration in meditation, and without this joy we wouldn't have enough fresh energy and creativity to continue on the path, to take care of our family, and to serve our society.

People in the helping professions, such as doctors, nurses, therapists, and social workers, can be burdened by the pain and suffering they're exposed to daily. I have met peace activists who have no peace or joy in themselves or in their views and outlook. Known as secondary trauma, this suffering of the pain of others is brought into our own body and mind.

In addition, we have our own worries, stress, unresolved pain, and unfinished business. These burdens accumulate in us, and even though our intention is good and noble, day-by-day we lose our freshness and joy; many of us become bitter, negative, and critical. We want to serve, and yet we may turn around and abuse those we're serving with harsh speech, unkind bodily actions, and negative thoughts of resentment, anger, blame, and judgment.

Mother's Pain

My mother was only in her early thirties, but she already had a lot of pain in her body. My mother would ask me, and my younger brother, to walk on her back. So we walked on her back as we were talking with each other.

At times I was thinking about other things, and I wasn't aware of my mother's body and her pain. I also wanted to get it over with so I could go play.

Years later, when I was in my early thirties, I started to develop pain in my joints and muscles. It became very frustrating to me. One day, while I was sitting quietly, an insight came to me.

"Insight" means to have light or sight into something that is mundane, something that you may have seen or experienced for years, but suddenly you see it as though for the first time.

This insight requires the day-to-day practice of awareness, so that after a process of gradual awakening, at a certain moment, the light is lit up suddenly.

So one day, as I was sitting quietly, I realized that I was experiencing my mother's pain. My mother passed away when I was twelve years old and more than twenty years had passed since then, but here I was experiencing her pain in my very own joints, in my very own muscles and in my very own body.

In that moment I felt deep connections and a deep intimacy that I had never before felt with my mother, even when she was still alive. My mother had never had time to stay home with us. She was always working, and then she died, so I never had moments of being close to her.

Yet here her body was, right inside my body, and I felt so close to her that the pain, her pain, became sacred to me. It was a joy to be with that pain, and it was no longer a burden. It was something in which I could connect and relate to my mother.

So where do you find joy? Where do you find what is sacred? In the ordinary things, in the mundane things, but we must be there in that moment to touch life deeply. Joy and the sacred are also found right there in the pain and the suffering that we experience.

Earth Is My Mother

When I came to the United States at the age of seventeen, I didn't speak much English except "How are you?" and "I am fine. Thank you." In high school one day, a young man in my English as a Second Language class asked me, "What are you doing?" I replied, "I am fine. Thank you!" Then, five minutes later, I realized what he had asked, and I was embarrassed for the whole day.

So I spent many years in school trying to learn English, finishing high school, going to college, and then to medical school. I didn't have time to pay attention to nature or to appreciate nature. I was fortunate that I had friends who loved nature and took me to the woods for hikes and for camping trips; those are the greatest gifts my friends have given me.

When I came to this practice, our Teacher continued to water that love of nature in me. In our community, our Sangha, many brothers and sisters also love nature, so we help each other to nourish and strengthen that seed in us.

Thay has spoken a lot about the Earth as our Mother and the Sun as our Father. I have learned to touch more deeply my love and appreciation for nature. Since I contracted Lyme disease, my energy level fluctuates greatly. I can be happy and joyful right now, and then the next minute I'm down and out; the energy is deflated.

When I'm too tired to continue and must lie down, I like to have the window curtains pulled aside so I can look out and see the sky and the trees. This helps me to remember that life continues to be there whether I'm sleeping or awake; whether I'm present or not present. Life continues to be there.

Life is very beautiful, and it's important to be reminded of that, to look out, to see the snow, and to say, "Mother, yet another beautiful coat, another beautiful dress you are putting on! Thank you for this gift."

Day after day, I learn to touch that beauty more and to touch that love more. When I lie down, I also learn to say to Mother Earth, "Please hold me. Hold this pain that I feel in my body. Help me to take care of it. Help me to accept it as it is."

In the moment you can entrust your pain and suffering to something greater than your body—however many pounds, feet, and inches it is—you no longer feel so lonely or caught. You don't dwindle in despair anymore. You know you can entrust and all will be okay, because life continues and you are a part of that life.

On this New Year's Eve, when the Sangha gathered in Blue Cliff's Great Harmony Meditation Hall and read our prayer to Mother Earth and Father Sun, an insight came to me.

Many years ago when, as a child I walked on my mother's back, I hadn't been aware of her body or her pain. However, now that I'm an adult, educated, sophisticated, and aware, I can no longer claim that excuse. Now, if I'm walking and I don't know that I am walking, I am still walking on my mother's back without the awareness that I am walking all over her, trampling on her, and causing her so much pain and damage.

This is true when we walk on Mother Earth as well.

The Earth is our mother. Some of us have never met our mother.

Some of us have lost our mother, when we were very young or when we were older. Even if you still have your mother with you, you may not be very pleased with her. You may not be able to forgive her unskillfulness or for the pain and sadness that she has transmitted to you.

Touch this great Mother Earth. Is she any less than our mother? How can one define a mother? What is a mother? She provides us everything—even our own body, our daily sustenance, the air that we breathe.

When we're born of our biological mother, the umbilical cord is cut, but with this Great Mother, the umbilical cord is never cut. We're still in her atmospheric embrace. If you are cut off from it, you can't breathe. So we're still in the womb of our Great Mother.

Can you touch that intimate connection? You don't have to touch it all the time, but if you come back to this awareness more and more often, then you will no longer feel so lonely and cut off. You wouldn't say, "Poor me, I don't have a mother!" "Poor me, I lost my father when I was very young," or "Poor me, my father is horrible."

In our spiritual life, we always have our mother and our father, and they are always there for us. At the moment I recognized that, I was still walking on my mother's back. I also realized that it's never too late to connect with her and heal her.

Back then, as a child, I wasn't aware of my mother's body and her pain, but now I can be aware of those things so that I can do my best to take care of her—to live as beautifully as I can, to live as peacefully as I can, to walk on her as gently and as mindfully as I can—so that someday I won't look back and regret, and especially at the last moment of my life, I won't have

Joy

to say, "I haven't lived my life. I haven't touched love in my life."

Many people in their dying moments actually cry out or scream. Those can be terrifying moments, with patients cursing at the doctors and nurses, screaming and yelling because they're so frightened. I have also seen patients lying there on their deathbed, looking at the door and waiting for someone to come, but nobody comes, not even their own partner or their own children. They're frightened and in deep despair.

Practicing, Studying, Working, and Playing

You may think that having a spiritual practice means that you scrutinize suffering under a microscope all the time. The truth is that cultivating joy is just as important as taking care of our suffering. A skilled gardener doesn't just pull weeds, but will also plant flowers and trees because when there are more flowers and trees, there's less space for the weeds to grow.

Many people are surprised to come to our practice centers and see monastic brothers and sisters smiling joyfully. They anticipate that monks and nuns are solemn and stern, but they see us always smiling. Children come to our monasteries all year long. Our brothers and sisters sing joyful practice songs, play hide-and-seek, and play sports with the children. Thay has taught us that as monastic practitioners, we need to pay equal attention to all four aspects of practicing, learning, working, and playing, and that we can also generate a lot of joy and happiness in these daily activities.

Playing is an important element, because playing and playfulness have the capacity to generate joy and happiness so that we can walk on this path our whole life.

In true practice, there is learning, working, and playing. One element includes all the other elements, in the true spirit of interbeing. Everyone needs a spiritual dimension in life. We practice mindfulness concretely through the practices of mindful breathing, mindful walking, mindful eating, sitting meditation, and so on, so that every aspect of our life can be in harmony and in balance.

Breathe, You Are Online

Students of all levels and ages can benefit greatly from the practice of mindfulness. During the twenty-four years that I was in school, every time I sat down to study or read a book, I would gnaw my nails down to my flesh, which bled, and when I washed my hands, the water touched the open wound and it would feel like an electric shock.

When I was in college, I would buy an expensive bitter liquid that was supposed to prevent you from biting the nails, but it tasted bitter only for a split second, and then I would still put my fingers into my mouth and chew them down with no problem because the habit energy was so strong.

Anxiety and stress associated with my study were so strong that often my fingers went into my mouth without me being aware of it. Now when I sit at the computer, I learn to follow my breathing. I can read an email or a book and follow my breathing at the same time. I can be typing and following my breathing at the same time. So I've trained myself to bring the element of practice into my studies, my work, and whatever I am doing, so that I don't inflict more pain upon my body and mind.

Thay has written a calligraphy that says, "Breathe, you are online."

This practice helps our mind to remain anchored in our body instead of being lost in the information and images on the computer screen. Many people download a bell of mindfulness onto their computer, so that they can stop every fifteen or thirty minutes in order to return to their breathing. Some programs even freeze the screen temporarily, and all you can do is to breathe and smile.

Warming Our Feet

While running, jogging, or playing with children, we can continue to follow our breathing, to be aware of the body and the movement of the body. As monastic practitioners, we have a chance to be children all over again. Perhaps I never had a chance to be a child before, because by the age of seven I'd already learned to take care of my brother while my mother went to work from early morning to late afternoon. There were nights my mother would go somewhere and would lock me inside the house. Thoughts about my childhood were often associated with loneliness, fear, confusion, and shame. Joyful moments, like the times my brother and I would put soap on the cement floor and slide back and forth, were much rarer.

Fortunately, in my relationships with my partners, they brought me to nature and helped me to cultivate my love for it and to touch deep appreciation and joy. Thay has also brought me close to nature. In our practice centers, we go for walking meditation in the woods every day. All of our monasteries are away from cities, and they're always in a natural environment surrounded by trees. This constant exposure to nature lightens up our thinking and softens our hearts. Consequently, friends coming to our practice centers for the first time feel calm and peaceful right away, even before they've had a chance to learn anything about the practice of mindfulness. That's also one main reason why we prefer to have retreats at our centers instead of somewhere else, such as a university campus or conference center.

Our practice is also friendly toward families and children. In playing with them and in playing with each other, our monastic brothers and sisters also become children because we don't have any sort of agenda or hidden motives. We can be carefree.

At Deer Park Monastery we have access to the Escondido mountain range, and on Lazy Days we would go hiking. We roamed together from morning to late afternoon. We sat on meadows of flowers. Whenever we liked, we'd sit down and enjoy the beautiful scenery and each other's company. We laughed and played in the fields. During one winter season, it was raining heavily and there was even thunder. We all put on our raincoats, went out into the rain and climbed up the waterfall. That day I had found a yellow safety hat left behind by a construction worker and I wore it because I was afraid that the hail would hit my head or the rain would get onto my glasses and I wouldn't be able to see. My brothers and sisters were laughing at the sight of me with the yellow safety hat.

Beautiful moments and joyful memories continue to nourish me. One time we went on a hike and we all got soaking wet, so we had to build a fire of broken branches to warm ourselves up. We took off our shoes and twisted water out of our socks, and held our feet near the fire. Our feet were blanched white like dead fish and wrinkled like raisins. One brother suddenly recited, "Warming our feet over the rosy hearth." It was a play on words from Thay's poem "Butterflies over the Golden Mustard Fields."

"Warming my hands over the rosy hearth, waiting for our evening meal, as the curtain of night falls slowly on our village." This is the image of a child waiting for his mother to finish cooking the evening meal; and meanwhile he's washing his feet and warming his hands over the fire.

As soon as my brother recited, "Warming our feet over the rosy hearth," all of us recognized that this came from our Teacher's poem and we laughed heartily.

Moments like this nourish us, allowing us to let go of everything—the past, worries, sadness, plans, and projects. Most of us that day were Dharma teachers, and yet our best moments were when we were being joyful and playful as children. In fact, being able to play together has helped our brothers and sisters understand each other at a deeper level and, as a result, we can let go of trivial conflicts more easily and work together harmoniously.

Before I was ordained, I had been perceived by others as pensive and serious. I was pursuing my career as a doctor, so I spent most of my time studying. Sometimes when I was sad or crying, if my partner smiled, I would think he was being insensitive or indifferent. I would reproach him, "How can you be smiling when I'm crying and saying these things to you?"

Now, as a nun, I will be the one to smile or make a joke to lighten up the moment when I feel there's tension or a heavy energy in a meeting or conversation. I have learned the value of humor and of joy.

Neuro-Lyme disease has also affected my personality in that it tends to make me more restless and less self-inhibited than before. Thanks to mindfulness, I'm able to relax my body and thoughts so I can remain calm and still for the most part. For example, during a meeting, certain goofy thoughts may arise, but I breathe and let them go because it would be inappropriate to blurt them out.

On the other hand, as I channel the energy of restlessness and disinhibition into that of joy, I sometimes do choose to blurt them out, especially when the atmosphere in the room is too serious.

Everyone laughs, especially when I add, "It's the tick that makes me say it!" My elder sister, Sister True Vow, would sometimes affectionately admonish me, "Now, don't you blame everything on the tick!"

As monastic practitioners, we're poor in terms of material possessions, but we're rich because we have time and space to discover ourselves and to be playful and happy. When I give orientation talks about our practice of mindful breathing, I often teasingly tell our lay friends that here in the monastery every time we hear the bell being invited, we stop everything that we're doing and return to our breathing. If we're speaking, we just let go of the rest of the sentence. If we're carrying something, we just put it down. If we're walking, we just stand still. We even let go of our thoughts and ideas. We simply enjoy our breathing in and out three times. In-breath and out-breath, that's one. In-breath and out-breath, that's two. In-breath and out-breath, that's three. So we breathe in three times and out three times.

In the monastery when we hear a phone ringing, we also breathe in and out three times like that, and then we walk mindfully to the phone. People who don't know about our practice may have hung up by the time we get to the phone, but that's okay, because if it's important, they'll call back and wait for us to pick up the phone. Those who know us will let the phone ring five or ten times, because they know we're taking our time to breathe and to walk, and they also have a chance to enjoy their breathing in the meantime. Out there, you may have a lot more money and ambition than we do, but you can't afford to breathe three times like us. So then maybe you can breathe in and out at least one time. I tease our lay friends with the hope of inspiring them to have a simple life, to know that they have enough, so that they can enjoy being themselves more.

A MILLIONAIRE WALKING

One of our lay practitioners is a millionaire who has been Thay's student for over twenty years. He shared with us that when he walks from his office to his secretary's office or to a meeting room, he sings silently to himself, "Breathing, smiling. Walking, happy." "Breathing, smiling. Walking, happy."

Before people come into the meeting room, he does slow walking in order to relax his body and quiet his mind. If there are other people around, he may walk a little faster because he doesn't want anyone to know that he's practicing, but he still keeps that tune in his mind, "Breathing, smiling. Walking, happy."

When people are speaking during the meeting, he listens quietly as he breathes in, closing his fingers into a gentle fist, and as he breathes out, opening his fingers and fist.

This is how he stays mindful of his breathing; he has seen our Teacher doing this and he has brought this practice into his daily life. So, while people are busy expressing their ideas and thoughts and arguing back and forth, this millionaire will sit there calmly, breathing-in, breathing-out, closing his hand, opening his hand, and smiling.

Toward the end of the meeting, inevitably people will turn around and ask him what he thinks, since he hasn't said a word. "When I finally speak," he told us, "everyone listens to me, and I usually have the best idea." Having been able to remain relaxed and calm during the entire meeting, he is able to listen deeply to all ideas and to synthesize them with clarity, wisdom, and innovation. This is the secret to his success, but he also adds that his true success has been his capacity to transform his suffering, and that he owes his life to the Dharma.

THIS IS A HAPPY MOMENT

In one Dharma talk, Thay told us that he has a new mantra, "This is a happy moment." Since then, every time we have a chance to sit down with Thay to drink tea or to share a meal, Thay would say, "This is a happy moment," and we would all smile in response. Sometimes Thay would ask, "What is this moment, my child?" and then a sister or a brother would smile and reply, "Dear Thay, this is a happy moment." It's a mantra, because when we pronounce it, we have mindfulness of our breathing and of our body.

This mindfulness, in turn, enables us to get in touch with the conditions of happiness that are available to us. As we say the mantra, it deepens our awareness of the happiness that is right here and right now for us.

A condition of happiness may be very simple. It is the presence of our beloved Teacher who is still with us in his familiar physical manifestation. It is the presence of our dear brothers and sisters who in the upcoming days may depart and go in the four directions. It may be the presence of your child, your partner, or your mother. It may be the blue sky, a birdsong, a purple flower by the sidewalk. It may simply mean that you can walk in this moment, and that your eyes can still see. These are all conditions of happiness that can nourish us and give us energy to walk joyfully together on this path.

The bodhisattvas, or great beings, have made the vow to walk the joyful path life after life with all living beings. All of us want to bring love to others and to offer our service to others, and we need to see ourselves as bodhisattvas, cultivating peace, joy, and freedom in ourselves so that we can offer it to others and can walk this beautiful path for a long time.

Thay has also said, "If you love one another, but you cause each other to cry every day, then that is not true love." When you look at your family members or the people you serve, and you only see work, responsibilities, resentment, and blaming, then you know your love has withered and is no longer true love. These signs should alert and alarm you to the present state of your relationship.

While I was living in a college dormitory, one of our resident assistants was going to get married and someone asked her, "How do you know if you love this person? How do you know if you will be with him for the rest of your life?"

She replied, "I know I still love him if every time I see him I can still be happy, and I still look forward to seeing him."

At the time, I didn't know what to make of her comment, but it has stayed with me all of these years. Now I have learned that love is organic, and so are passion and joy. You can't rely on these fleeting feelings for confirmation of your love. If they change into something else, such as hatred, anger, or resentment, you and your partner may walk away from each other.

Yet, because everything is organic, we can learn to transform this kind of negativity back to awareness, gratitude, joy, and happiness. Everything needs food to survive. The capacity to be truly present enables us to touch joy and love in our daily life. Indeed, every interaction can be a love story. Every person, flower, and pebble can be our beloved.

WAVES ARE LAUGHTER

There is a wonderful poem about generating joy:

> Let's generate cloud and sunshine.
> Generate it for yourself and do not borrow
> from the earth and the sky,
> so that when the sun and the moon are still far away,
> on the front porch, moonlight continues to shine.

This poem is also a beautiful practice: generating cloud and sunshine in one's own heart.

Since the time I was a child, I have found solace in singing. Sometimes I would feel so saddened and lost, and so I walked on the street and sang made-up songs to myself. I would sing about what was happening in that day or what was happening in my life. Singing became a constant companion to me and it soothed my pain.

Many people liked my singing, but they often commented that it was heartwrenching, and it made them feel saddened and uneasy.

As a matter of fact, my sadness was so deep that it expressed itself even while I was chanting and inviting the great temple bell. One time, an elder sister came to me and suggested that I shouldn't invite the great temple bell for a while. The sound of the temple bell travels a great distance, and it's supposed to awaken all beings in the ten directions, including those in the hell realm. She said that my sad chanting voice along with the sound of the bell may neither help to inspire these beings nor liberate them.

I cried when my elder sister told me not to invite the temple bell for a while, but I understood her message. I also recognized that when I sang and chanted in Vietnamese, my voice sounded saddest. My singing and chanting in English sounded less sad, because I had learned English in the United States and because I had also learned to be more confident in myself and to experience more conditions of happiness than when I was a child.

When I went to France to ordain as a nun, I also learned some French and, amazingly enough, there was no sadness in my voice when I sang in French, because at that time I already knew the practice and had begun to transform my suffering.

Therefore, the language that we use and the sounds of music that we produce can manifest our deep consciousness. Whether it's joy or sadness or anger, it will be expressed in our speech, in our lyrics, and in our music. Thus, we practice to speak more lovingly and we use practice songs to water the seeds of happiness and joy in us.

Now when Thay hears me sing, he joyfully exclaims, "Your voice is not sad anymore!" This is a great compliment to me.

About a year ago, I had a memorable dream. I was standing peacefully on the shore, and the waves were high and roaring. I saw my Teacher in the distance, and he was walking toward me. Then he turned to walk into the ocean, and so did I. At that moment, my body dissolved into the water. My Teacher was also no longer separated from the water. There were only the ocean and the waves, and a roaring laughter above the waves. A thought arose from this enmeshed consciousness, "Waves are the laughter of the ocean." That laughter was like the last physical manifestation of me before it, too, melted into the ocean. I woke up with a deep sense of joy and oneness.

Chapter Four

TRUST AND CONFIDENCE

Without faith it is not possible for human beings to live. Without love
we cannot fully realize our full humanity. We practice the Dharma not
only to gain knowledge but to transform ourselves into someone who is
capable of love, affection, and gratitude.

—Thich Nhat Hanh, *Peaceful Action,*
Open Heart: Lessons from the Lotus Sutra

TRUST IN BUDDHA NATURE

According to Webster's dictionary, faith means "a strong belief or trust."
Trust means, "to have a strong belief in the goodness or in the ability
of someone or something." And confidence is "a feeling or belief that
you can do something well or succeed at something." The words faith,
trust, and confidence are often used interchangeably. Among the several
Sanskrit words for trust and confidence, I have chosen the word vishvas,
which includes not only the meanings of trust and confidence but also the

consequences that those elements bring: breathing freely, freedom from fear, confidence, reliance, comfort, encouragement, and inspiration.

Faith or trust is an essential element in the Buddhist teachings and practices. For example, the Five Powers are faith, diligence, mindfulness, concentration, and insight. These are the five faculties that each person inhabits intrinsically, but when we practice these five faculties they can become powers in us. Faith can be referred to as faith in oneself—in one's capacity to wake up, to heal, to transform, to be the most beautiful, wholesome, and true person that one can possibly be. We also have faith in the Dharma, in the teachings and the practices that enable us to realize the Buddha nature in us. We have faith in the Sangha, the community of practitioners who give us guidance and support on the path of practice.

Often we have faith in something before we really know what it is. When we were children, we didn't know anything about soap, but our parents told us, "You should wash your hands every time you go to the bathroom or before you go into the kitchen." Following their guidance, we washed our hands and saw that our hands became cleaner, and so we developed faith in soap, and from that experience we've continued to use soap daily.

Some of us may embark on a spiritual journey because we see our grandparents, our parents, or other people practicing and they have good results, so we follow their example. Some of us come to a practice center without knowing anything about the Buddha's teachings and practices, but we've heard about it from other people. So we give ourselves a chance to come to the practice center and begin to practice; it's only been a few days, but we already feel the peace, the calm, the clarity, and the relaxation in our body and mind. It makes us want to practice more deeply because we directly experience the results of our practice. Only when we have this faith, are we able to continue the practice with diligence and tenacity.

In the Kalama Sutra, the Buddha taught his disciples and the Brahmans who came to ask him for advice not to believe blindly in his teachings, or in the claims anyone else makes, because that person is famous, espousing a known view, or because the majority is following it. We have to experiment with it, practice it, and apply it, in our daily life, and then we can see the direct results. If it works, then that is when we can truly believe in something. So we don't believe blindly or have faith out of desperation.

Sometimes from desperation we also try to find something to hold onto, something to save us, like looking for a float when we're drowning. For example, when we've lost a loved one, we experience some trauma; or our loved ones undergo a major crisis, we may turn to religion in order to find comfort and hope. This temporary assistance and relief can be helpful. However, it's our daily application of the practice that makes our faith strong, enduring, and real to us. Faith in oneself and in one's path will enable one to have faith in other people—faith that they, too, have the capacity to heal physically and mentally, to be their most beautiful, wholesome, and true, and to be able to walk on the same path together with us.

In true love, we must have trust and confidence in each other. This is a practice not of spontaneous feeling, but of concrete daily observations of ourselves and of each other.

Thay has shared with us, his monastic disciples, that his teacher always trusted him and had confidence in him; and that has been his deep happiness and nourishment. As our Teacher, Thay has also entrusted in us his utmost trust and confidence. On the day of my ordination, I knelt next to Thay, joined my palms and said to him, "Respected Thay, I promise that I will practice wholeheartedly in order to deserve to be your disciple." He smiled ever so gently and told me, "Thay has full confidence that you will practice successfully, and that you will help many people."

Over the years, in my darkest moments of despair, I would think of Thay or he would appear in my dreams, and my being would be imbued with his sense of love and trust. If you fall down many times in your life, you may begin to lose faith in yourself and in your capacity to transform and to heal. Thus, it's a great blessing to be loved and trusted by someone else, especially by your teacher, by your parents, by your partner or friend. Then, in loving them and in trusting them, you learn to love and trust yourself. This is a great gift that we can practice to give to ourselves and to offer to our beloved.

From my Teacher's example, I have also done my best to instill trust and confidence in others, by acknowledging their positive qualities, talents, and actions, and by encouraging them to use the mindfulness practice to overcome their complexes and difficulties.

SPACIOUSNESS

Each one of us needs to have a spiritual dimension in our life so that we may actively transform and heal ourselves in our daily life. Knowing that the other person is also doing the same thing, we can have trust and confidence in him or in her. Naturally, trust brings respect, and vice versa. Trusting that each one of us is taking good care of ourselves, for our own sake, for each other's sake, and for the sake of the world, we respect each other's time and space to do this.

When I think of my Teacher, I only need to smile and breathe because I know that he is smiling and breathing mindfully right now. It also makes me happy to know that my brothers and sisters are doing the same thing that I am doing, which is cultivating mindfulness in everything we do. This gives me a sense of peace and assurance about the ones I love and trust. It helps remove the need to be next to somebody, to receive the acknowledgement, the praise, or the attention of that person so that I can feel secure.

When we find ourselves always in need of another person's time and space and attention, it's most likely because we aren't giving that to ourselves. So we intrude on the space, time, and freedom of the other person, and sooner or later, we become weary of one another, and we become disappointed and dissatisfied. We have to meet these needs for ourselves so that the coming together of two people doesn't happen out of loneliness, neediness, unrealistic expectations or perceptions, or imagined fantasies that we have of each other; but so that it comes from a place that we feel whole and that we have something to offer to each other and learn from each other.

Sometimes we may see ourselves as incomplete, then we look for the other half to complete ourselves, but that usually makes us even more needy, insecure, and full of expectations. However, if we develop ourselves as a whole person, and we're comfortable being with ourselves, quietly listening to ourselves, accepting what was, what is, and what will be in our lives, then when we come together with somebody else, it's from a place of spaciousness and freedom. We will know how to appreciate and protect the space, time, and freedom of another person, doing everything we can to help that person cultivate his or her own freedom.

In my past relationships with my partners, I was fortunate to be able to trust them completely. Thanks to my ancestors, the tendency to have doubt and suspicion is minimal in me. In fact, I tend to trust people unless they behave poorly. My partners also earned my trust by being supportive and loving and proper in every way. When we met up with friends, we would enjoy speaking with different groups of friends without the need to be seen together all the time. I remember one time I saw from a distance that a friend of my best friend was talking to my partner, and it was quite clear that she was being flirtatious with him. Out of amusement and curiosity I sat silently and watched them. My partner was proper and polite to her, but not in any way did he joke back or try to do anything to respond to her flirtatious behavior. At one point, she turned around to get some more drinks, and he immediately stood up to walk toward me and then sat down next to me. I trusted my partners in every way, and I could go to India, Japan, Kenya, or Vietnam for almost three months on each trip with the complete confidence that they would take the best care of themselves and of our relationship.

My partners had their own hobbies and projects and other things that they loved to do. They could be comfortable with themselves, and they had their own circle of positive friends. So in that way I could feel free to be myself and to do whatever I needed to do without having to suffer from any sort of insecurity or worry that they would behave inappropriately in my absence. I also treated my partners with respect and behaved appropriately, so they also felt comfortable to be themselves and to trust me. This mutual trust enabled our relationships to deepen at every level, and enabled us to live our lives more deeply as individuals and as a couple.

The Buddha taught about the emptiness of transmission: that the transmitter, the receiver, and the object of transmission are in each other, that they are each other. We can apply this to true love. In true love, the lover, the beloved, and the love are not three separate entities. They are in each other. The lover is the beloved. The lover is the love. To love oneself is to love one's beloved. To learn to trust oneself is to learn to trust one's beloved. It's in this process of loving and trusting that we discover ourself and our beloved. So these three elements are intimately woven together.

With trust and confidence in each other and in our relationship, we can be bodhisattvas for each other—enlightened beings who have made the great vow to help other beings go through suffering and attain happiness and liberation. Sometimes we're caught in our roles as partners, as spouses, as parents, or as children. We perform these roles mechanically, while we harbor an underlying disappointment and bitterness that's built up over the years as a result of unskillful speech, behavior, and actions. In the beginning the relationship was so bright and beautiful, and then with time it becomes laden with so much unskillfulness that we simply learn to endure one another.

But as bodhisattvas on the joyful path, we recognize that we have made the vow to be together and help each other realize the fullest potential of our Buddha nature. Then we're responsible for our karma, including our bodily actions, speech, and thoughts, and we help the other person to transform, heal, and refine their bodily actions, speech, and thoughts, their suffering and difficulties. We won't be so quick to blame one another. A relationship is a long process, and it can be a joyful and meaningful process when we have the spiritual practice to support one other.

In the Vietnamese tradition, there are two elements to love; one is *tinh* and the other is *nghia*. Tình can be understood as the infatuation, passion, or desire that two new lovers may have for one another. As time passes, the romance or desire will no longer be the most important aspect in their life together. It will settle down like dust in the sprinkling rain. Then it's in our daily support of each other, it's in our daily discovery of each other that we build a deeper relationship, as if we were brothers and sisters of each other, as if we were parents of each other. This is nghia, the deep love and support for each other that helps us overcome any obstacles and difficulties that arise. New love is like a seed that you've just planted, but you're already envisioning the flowers, the fruits, and the harvest. In true love, the two trees have grown wide and deep roots into the earth and their roots are intertwined and enmeshed into one solid foundation.

INHERITANCE IN THE PATH

Prince Siddhartha was married and had a child. His wife Yasodhara was also his soul mate who listened to him and understood his desire to be free. When he wanted to become an ascetic to seek the path, she let him go and she didn't try to stop him. She pretended to be asleep, so that he could leave quietly, and his father and the guards wouldn't know. When he became enlightened, the Buddha came back to visit his father, his son, and his former wife. Yasodhara stood silently looking at him from the balcony. Then she told their son, Rahula, "Ask your father for your inheritance." So the young child approached the Buddha and asked for his inheritance. In that moment, Yasodhara not only trusted the Buddha, his vision, and his path, but now she also entrusted her only child to him. The inheritance to his son lay in the monastic robe. The inheritance to his son is the Path. The Buddha wouldn't have jewels or kingdoms to pass on to his son, but the Buddha had the life of enlightenment to transmit to his son.

Soon after that visit, Rahula followed the Buddha to become the youngest monk in the Sangha, and later he also became enlightened. Yashodhara's absolute love and trust also enabled her to leave her comfortable position as a princess later on in order to follow the path and become a nun and achieve enlightenment herself. Therefore, the love and trust that we have in each other enable us to let go of many attachments and expectations and open up a whole new dimension in our life as in the case of Yasodhara, Rahula, and Prince Siddhartha.

PRISONER OF DISTRUST

There are situations in which people say, "I love him, but I don't trust him," or, "I love her, but I don't trust her." When you hear yourself saying that, it should be a bell of mindfulness. You should look deeply into the nature of your love, because love without trust is not true love. Perhaps it's out of insecurity or out of grasping that we're holding on to each other, so the relationship continues even though there's no trust in it. I know some young teenage girls, even women and men, who stay in a relationship while their partner, husband, or wife has affairs or other relationships. They still hold on to this relationship because they fear that if they let go of it nobody else will love them; they may not be able to find someone else to be with.

Once a young man asked me sincerely, "Do you believe in true love?" He wanted to become a monk and that was one of his main concerns. I said to him, "Yes, I believe in true love. Unfortunately, most of us settle for sex and security." Security could be financial security or just having someone next to you so that you don't feel lonely or afraid. We may lack the capacity and the trust that we can be with ourselves and take care of ourselves, so we look for another person to be with us and to take care of us. Unfortunately, we often meet up with someone who is in the exact same dilemma; two lonely and distrusting people only make the loneliness and distrust exponentially greater.

In a relationship, people may have layers of pain, betrayal, distrust, or jealousy that have been building up over the years. They remain together but they don't forgive each other.

Recently I met a couple who were on retreat. The man was literally begging for his wife's forgiveness and attention. He was already in his sixties, but the way his eyes looked at her was like the eyes of a child yearning for his mother's love, attention, and forgiveness. The wife remained standoffish and cold, withholding her physical affection from him and standing at a distance with her arms crossing her chest. If he tried to touch her, her body would stiffen. I don't know if he had betrayed her when he was younger, but I could see that both of them were in deep pain.

The thought that arose in me was: let go of this relationship and let go of each other; but if you stay together, then let go of the old hurt. You can't have both, because you will only hurt each other so much more. It was painful to watch them, and I tried to help them to reconcile with each other. She was in a lot of physical pain, and both of them were aware that this pain came from her holding on to this tension and resentment for so many years. When I hugged her, her body was stiff and rigid like a pillar of metal.

I thought about their old age. All he wanted was for them to live peacefully together in their old age. They had already struggled so hard in their youth to raise a family and to have status in society. Now they had everything, and what was most important to him was that he and his wife could be happy and peaceful together. If they didn't practice to transform and heal the old pain, they would continue to hurt each other for the remaining days of their lives; they wouldn't be able to rest in peace, to let go of their bodies, or to let go of each other.

In learning to trust each other, we must help each other cultivate a spiritual dimension in our lives in order to transform our wounds and heal them from within. We have a beautiful practice of Beginning Anew in which we come back to ourselves, recognizing the positive things in ourselves and the good efforts that we've made in our lives. We also water the flowers in our partner, expressing our appreciation for their positive qualities and actions. Then the second step is to express our own regret. One partner may say, "I'm sorry. I was young and irresponsible, but I didn't mean to hurt you. I pray and hope that you are well. Please forgive me and please help me to forgive myself."

This is a practice of loving speech, speaking with utmost sincerity and humility to ourselves and to the other person. We put aside our pride and arrogance, taking responsibility for our own actions. It's helpful to speak clearly, slowly, and gently. When a wave of emotion surges, we simply return to our breathing to calm it down before we resume speaking. Loving speech helps open the door to our own hearts and to the other person's heart. People may justify speaking harshly by claiming that they're only saying what they feel is right or true, and that's just the way they are. However, we all know too well that this kind of talk only puts up walls between our loved ones and ourselves. As soon as one person begins to speak, the other person already assumes that he or she knows what will be said next.

Sometimes we may also refuse to share our feelings or to explain ourselves to the other person, expecting that he or she should already know our feelings or intentions. This attitude can lead to further separation and misunderstanding. Loving speech enables deep listening to take place; we hear not only what is said but also what is underneath all those words. Awareness of breathing helps us to keep our mind quiet and spacious and filled with equanimity, releasing our own internal commentaries and arguments, so that we can be truly present for the other person's sharing. When we agree or disagree with what's being said, we're not giving ourselves the chance to gain a deeper understanding of the other person, because those agreements and disagreements are already our own preconceptions and attitudes. We simply listen so that the other person may have a chance to release the tension and suffering resulting from having hung onto certain experiences, perceptions, and views.

The practice of deep listening takes place in our daily practice of sitting meditation, in which we learn to be there for ourselves, listening to our own breathing, body, thoughts, views, and perceptions without giving preferences or having judgments toward them. In deep listening, we may hear for the first time what has been said one hundred or one thousand times before. A son may say to his mother, "Is this what you mean, Mother?" or you may say to yourself, "Is this what you've been trying to tell me all these years, my own heart?"

Perhaps it's most difficult to forgive ourself for having been the main perpetrator and the prison guard of our own suffering. We can acknowledge that we didn't know a better way to think, to behave, and to speak. Therefore, we committed unwholesome actions toward ourselves and others. Now we have a concrete spiritual practice to help us not to repeat those mistakes and to help prevent others from making that same mistake. When we actively do that, we can forgive ourselves. So it isn't forgetting about what happened, as though you have amnesia about something in the past, but it's because you know that you have a path, that you are doing it better now, and this confidence brings about forgiveness toward yourself. If the other person is still alive, you can write a letter to that person or ask to speak to them. If that person is dead or can't be contacted, you can always do Beginning Anew with that person inside of you, because every experience that you go through is never lost. That person has become an intricate part of you.

In our society, people quickly resort to divorce because they believe that once they're separated or divorced, it will be the end of their problems. Looking deeply, we will see the truth is that the person can never be separated or divorced from us. Even if that person is not biologically related to us, the experiences that we had together will always be there in our consciousness, and we continue to live with that person in our consciousness.

A few years after I became a nun, I had a chance to visit with Patrick, and he told me, "You know, sometimes when I'm driving I still find myself arguing with you." I laughed, but I felt a deep pang of pain. Out of unskillfulness I had blamed him for not understanding me and my sadness. He did his best, but my expectations were unreasonable. Now as a nun, I told him, "Please forgive me. Whatever points or arguments I tried to make, I was wrong, so please let go of them and don't argue with me anymore." In our relationship, sometimes we just want to be right. We become righteous and we're willing to sacrifice our love and respect for each other, so that we can prove ourselves to be right. Unfortunately, this wounds each one of us deeply. In our practice of Beginning Anew, what we cherish above all is the harmony within our body and mind and between us, the lover and the beloved. For the sake of harmony, we reconcile so that we can have peace and stability in ourselves, in each other, and in the relationship. If one person would say, "What coud I have said or done that would make it better?" the other person could already breathe more easily. Rights or wrongs, they are simply relative, situational, and not absolute.

JEALOUSY AND ENVY

As I said in the beginning, wherever there are oak trees, there are also rocks and boulders. Over the years, an oak might grow over the rock and into the rock, and its deep roots would be woven with the rock in the earth. The rock and the oak, they are two, but they have become one. They support each other. The rock offers the stability and the minerals to the oak, and the oak stands tall but deeply rooted in the earth and in the rock.

When we make the commitment to share a path, we must be able to grow in our love, our transformation, and our healing in the spirit of the rock and the oak. Your happiness is my happiness, and your suffering is my suffering. Taking care of me is taking care of you, and taking care of you is taking care of me. Then we won't have issues such as jealousy, which is the opposite of trust and confidence. As partners or spouses, we can be jealous of each other. We may think that our partner is more interested in other people than in us, and we experience insecurity, envy, or jealousy. A young man in a Dharma sharing session shared in front of his wife and everybody,

"Sister, in your presence I would like to share that I am a very proper man. I love my wife and my son, but I don't know why my wife keeps saying things to me as if she doesn't trust me. She would always ask me where did I go or why did I come home late or who was I with today? The things she says to me are very painful."

I advised the young woman not to water the seed of mistrust in him and in herself. If it's true that he's proper in all his behaviors and you continue to be suspicious of him, then you know it's because you had been wounded earlier in life. Maybe you observed this inappropriate behavior in your own parents or in your past relationships. Then you need to acknowledge the source of your insecurity and suspicion, so that you can transform your wound. If your husband is truly loyal to you, but you keep making these insinuations and watering his seed of betrayal, then maybe he will become disloyal one day. We can turn somebody who is clean into an alcoholic, a drug addict, or a betrayer. If we ourselves are insecure, jealous, and full of suffering, then our way of thinking, speaking, and behaving can cause that person so much unnecessary stress, confusion, guilt, and weariness that they may become exactly what we're accusing them of. So it's important that we practice selective watering, recognizing and encouraging only the goodness in each other. When we see something negative, we can use loving speech and speak with humility and sincerity to help each other to transform.

Husbands and wives may be jealous of each other's talents and success, because they see their happiness as an individual matter. The other person may have a better job, make a better salary, have more talents, or get more attention at work, so then you feel insecure or jealous and this is detrimental to a relationship. In some situations, you see your partner losing a job, not being able to get a decent job, or not being able to succeed in what he or she is doing, and then you start to compare him or her to your friends' partners and you behave unkindly and disrespectfully toward your partner.

Jealousy can occur at different levels. Sometimes jealousy can manifest between parents and children. At the age of forty, my brother got married and had a child—a beautiful girl named Sunee, which means "a good thing" in Thai. Sunee was only four months old, but already there was some conflict in his marriage. He felt that he loved his daughter more than his wife now. He also felt that his wife should love him and Sunee more than her own mother and siblings. He jokingly told me his wife prioritized Sunee as first, her blood family as second, her dog as third, and him as fourth.

It was a joke because his wife didn't have a dog, but a joke does reflect the person's attitude. I was surprised to see this envy and jealousy in my brother, because all his life he was generous and loving. Unfortunately, in relationships we can easily become jealous and envious when our sense of self and what belongs to the self are most at stake.

I asked my brother to recall the time his wife was pregnant. She developed diabetes during pregnancy. Her life was at risk during her pregnancy and during the process of giving birth to his daughter. He owes that gratitude to her. To love Sunee is to cherish and love his wife even more. To love Sunee is to cherish and love her mother and siblings even more. I reminded my brother that I had asked my partners never to make me choose between them or my brother, because they would lose. I also gave my brother an acronym to practice with, "FAAR," which means flow as a river. Be generous. Be kind. Be supportive of her decisions.

When we don't have the insight and the practice of interbeing, we also suffer from separation and isolation. We compare ourselves to other people, and we revolve in the three complexes of inferiority, superiority, and equality. We don't have the insight of interbeing, that whatever qualities other people may have, those elements are also in us.

All mental states, known as mental formations in Buddhist psychology, exist in every one of us. Because of our individual life experiences, they may manifest differently, but we all have each of those mental formations. When we don't understand what we're made of, when we don't yet know how to love ourselves and to value harmony and healing, then we're willing to put ourselves up for auction, parading, "Hey, I'm better than you," "I'm equal to you," or "I'm less than you." There's insecurity and low self-esteem, and we feel the need to compete or to put somebody down so that we can feel a little better.

However, if we learn to love ourselves and take good care of ourselves, we will never have the need to put ourselves up for auction, or to put somebody else up for auction. The insight of interbeing can heal these three complexes that most of us experience—inferiority, superiority, and equality. Although equality in terms of fairness and justice is something good, it can also be a complex when we're caught in comparing ourselves to others, forgetting that we inter-are.

In my monastic life, I might recognize that some sisters are talented or good at certain things, and a thought might arise, "Ah, she is better than me!" There is a twinge of envy or jealousy, and I have learned to recognize it as soon as it arises.

In that moment, I have a choice. I can build up the envy and jealousy with additional negative thoughts and start to hate that person, try to compete with her, or put her down so I can feel better about myself. Or, in that very same instant, I also have a choice to recognize the thought as it is, breathe and smile to it, and then simply let it go because I know that it's wrong view and wrong thinking.

The quickest way to deal with these thoughts is to breathe, smile, and let go. Sometimes a thought can be persistent or perhaps our practice is still weak, so even though we recognize the thought as discriminative and skewed, other negative thoughts still build up quickly. When that happens, we can replace those negative thoughts with the more positive thoughts.

For example, I can give rise to the thought, "She is my sister, and I'm happy that she's talented because then she can help share joy and the Dharma with many other people."

Or I give rise to the image of Avalokiteshvara Bodhisattva who has a thousand hands and a thousand eyes so she can help many living beings. If there were only one hand and one eye, the work would be limited.

I can also feel love and empathy for myself, because I'm putting my body and mind through the stress of jealousy and envy. I have had the opportunity to obtain a higher education and to develop many talents, and if I still feel uncomfortable with someone who is more skilled than me, then it must be even more difficult and challenging for those who have had less opportunity in life. I also appreciate deeply Thay's teaching that the greatest talent is to be able to live in harmony with ourselves and with one another.

The image of the Great Being, Avalokiteshvara, and the desire to practice nondiscrimination guide me and give me the feeling of joy. In Vietnamese we call it *tuy hy*, which means you are happy with the happiness of another person, and you rejoice in the joy of another person; this joy is also known as the quality of mudita in true love. Husbands and wives can be envious or jealous of each other's success or of the attention that the other is receiving. Parents can feel insecure when their children advance to a high level in their career. Envy and jealousy can cause us to become unkind, unsupportive, and distant with our loved ones. Thus, we practice with it again and again every time it arises.

We can look deeply into our own life to understand these seeds of envy, jealousy, and separateness. Perhaps we didn't receive enough recognition, or we weren't listened to or understood as children, so we always felt insecure. If somebody gets more attention, we aren't able to accept that.

Perhaps the seed of jealousy or envy is strong in our ancestors, including our mother and father, and they have transmitted that seed to us, so we have their tendency to react to somebody who is more talented, more popular, or more loved than we are.

With the insight of interbeing and nondiscrimination between you and the other person, feelings of jealousy and separation can evaporate. This realization helps me to be more humble, empathetic, and supportive toward others. Gradually, I learn to see all of my monastic and lay brothers and sisters as the one thousand hands and one thousand eyes of the Bodhisattva, helping each other and other people.

I am not so discreet and skillful, unfortunately, so every so often I find myself causing some of my sisters to feel uncomfortable and hurt. When I went back to Plum Village to receive the Lamp Transmission to become a Dharma teacher in 2008, I was surprised to see that two of my younger sisters consistently avoided me. They never greeted me, and every time they saw me, they just turned the other way. I had never met them in person before, but I had heard that they were extremely intelligent, talented, and active in the Sangha.

During one Day of Mindfulness, I felt nauseated and achy all over my body. While I was resting in the Buddha Hall in the brothers' hamlet, I saw one of these two younger sisters. I walked up to her, smiled, and asked if she would kindly give me a massage. She looked astounded at first, but she agreed to it. After she massaged me for a few minutes, I could feel her becoming more relaxed and at ease and her touch more attentive and tender. Although we didn't speak to each other afterward, her energy seemed softer toward me for the rest of the time I was there. When I met her on the next teaching tour with Thay, she talked to me at times and even thanked me for cleaning the toilets regularly at the temple where we were staying. During this three-week stay in Plum Village for my lamp transmission, Thay also confided in me one day at his hermitage, "Thay is always kind. Still, there have been people accusing Thay of many things. Thay has remained silent, not trying to justify himself, and continued to do what he believes in . . . You cannot accomplish much alone. You should have at least two or three soul mates who understand you and share your ideals. Then you can realize your visions together."

In living together, my sisters have taught me to be more grateful, modest, and aware of myself and of others. I have also learned to allow myself to be more fragile and vulnerable to my sisters, asking them for help and support, so that we may have the opportunity to connect with each other at a level that is more humble and real.

TRANSITIONS AND TRESPASSES

Many of us may be looking to be in a relationship especially when we are pressured, lonely, restless, or when it's simply our habitual pattern. Many young women share that as they were growing up they observed their single mothers always in relationships, so they also began to be in relationships from the time they were teenagers, and they have never been out of a relationship since. Before the old one ended, the new one had already begun, and these transitions become a blur for many of them.

In our daily practice, we train ourselves to pay attention to every transition. As a part of our mindful manners, before we enter the restroom, we knock on the door three times, slowly and clearly. One time I asked my Teacher, "If you know that nobody is in the restroom, do you still need to knock on the door?" Thay replied, "How can you be so sure? There may be other beings in there." Since then I have always knocked on the door before I walk into the restroom.

Before I enter a room from the outside, I also stop at the threshold and breathe. When I enter the meditation hall, I pause to acknowledge that I am entering a sacred space,

> Entering the meditation hall,
> I see my true self.
> As I sit down,
> I vow to cut off all afflictions.

The meditation hall is sacred because my mind is fully present. I may simply give rise to the thought that this is a sacred space and may I protect this sacred space. Without mindfulness, one can walk into the meditation hall casually and noisily and having forgotten to first take off their shoes.

Often we barge into a space without being aware that the place may be quiet and we're talking loudly and disturbing the peace of that space. The place may also be full of people talking loudly, and if you're lost in your thoughts while you're walking into that space, their restless energy can affect you right away, and you may feel discombobulated or disoriented. So the energy of the place can affect us, and our energy can affect the energy of the place and the people, positively or negatively.

Therefore, it's important that we're in touch with our energy, so that we remain whole and stable as we make our daily transitions. This practice can be applied when we put on or take off our shoes, open the door, go into a car, leave the car, walk into our office, or enter our home. Being fully aware that we're returning home, we can choose to leave behind the worries and anxieties from work so that we can be fresh and new for our loved ones.

When we can't be aware of the physical transitions that we make in our daily life, we may also find ourselves not being aware at all of the transitions and trespasses that we make in our relationships. For example, you are still in a relationship, and you already find yourself spending time with somebody else; this can bring a lot of suffering and confusion to yourself, to your partner, and to the new person.

We can look at betrayal as a wave, just like a wave of thoughts, emotions, or perceptions. The moment we find out that somebody has betrayed us or that we have betrayed somebody is not the moment that betrayal takes place. A wave doesn't start at the peak or at the trough, but the wave has already begun much earlier when it was still underneath the surface of the ocean, and it has worked up its momentum until it manifests into a wave.

Daily mindful consumption—what we take in through our six senses—and daily awareness of our thoughts, speech, and bodily actions can help us to realize when our mind has begun to become bored with our present relationship, when we want to run away from problems and difficulties and take refuge in someone else or fantasize about another person. We need to detect those early signs and symptoms and reestablish communication with ourselves and with each other in order to avoid betraying ourselves, our partner, and our children.

GAME OF PURSUIT

Some people may pursue others as a game. You would do everything you can to get the person's attention. Once the person is paying attention to you or falling in love with you, then you find yourself feeling afraid, losing interest, or walking away simply because it gives you a sense of self-worth and importance. These are behavioral patterns of a wounded child. You are betraying yourself and the other person, and you cannot be happy when you no longer believe in true love.

Many of us are actually stuck in this sort of game. We must come back and take care of the wounded child within, because our inner child needs the love and attention that he or she never received. When we learn to offer affection and care to ourselves, we don't have to impose pain on each other anymore. One man shared that he played this game of pursuit for many years, and it was tiring. After every brief and exciting affair, he realized that he had to come back and face his own loneliness and restlessness. It was but a temporary distraction to pursue somebody; and you can never be entirely distracted from yourself. The child in you continues to cry out even if you try to stifle his or her voice.

I DON'T SLEEP WITH MY TEETH

Two men were talking to each other, and one man said, "You know, last night I couldn't sleep because my tooth hurt so much. Does that ever happen to you?"

This man was asking for some empathy. However, the other man replied, "I don't sleep with my teeth so I don't have that problem." That is a simple happiness right there. You still have teeth to sleep with!

From the third and fourth exercises of mindful breathing—"Breathing in, I am aware that I have a body. Breathing out, I am aware that I have a body. Breathing in, I calm my body. Breathing out, I relax my body."—we have the practice of Deep Relaxation. This is a favorite practice for practitioners of all ages. When I work with teenagers, I always offer a session of Deep Relaxation before Dharma sharing in the afternoon, and at the end of the last evening activity. They are not aware that they need rest, but most, if not all of them, sleep soundly during the session.

Our Teacher has often said that allowing yourself to rest after lunch is the most civilized thing to do. If you have an office, you can bring a mat, spread it out on the floor, and lie down to rest, even if it is for only five or ten minutes. You can find a quiet corner in a garden or in the building where you're working, or simply sit on a chair or a bench with your back leaning against the wall.

The first part of Deep Relaxation is to scan through the parts of your body, from your head to your toes, and relax each part with your mindful breathing and with your smile. For example, "Breathing in, I am aware of my head. Breathing out, I relax my head. I relax all the thoughts and feelings that are arising. Breathing in, I am aware of my forehead. Breathing out, I relax the vertical and horizontal lines on my forehead with a smile. Breathing in, I am aware of my gray hair. Breathing out, hello my dear gray hair. Breathing in, I am aware of my teeth. Breathing out, I smile to this non-toothache moment!"

As you scan through each internal and external organ, you can also send gratitude and affection to it. For example, "Breathing in, I am aware of my lungs. Breathing out, I smile to my lungs. Thank you for being there and working constantly. I have been unkind to you because I talk too much or I have been smoking for too many years. I am sorry, my dear. Please help me to take better care of you and to heal you." It may seem strange at first to communicate with your body, but your body is a living organism, and it is always communicating with you.

You can make it a good habit to scan your body regularly throughout the day. You will gain a deep appreciation for your body and for your life. You know that if you were to get into a car accident or to come down with a serious illness, the very ordinary things that you have now would mean everything. You would just want to be able to open your eyes, move your hands, breathe on your own, and walk on your own.

Similarly, if you remember that your beloved may depart tomorrow, you will naturally want to let go of all your worries, judgments, and expectations. You will want to cherish these last moments with him or her.

CHASING AFTER NOVELTY

Through our daily practice of self-love, self-understanding, living simply, and knowing that we have enough, we gradually transform our mind of desire and grasping.

Before I became a nun, when I went shopping I would be excited about the new clothes and the new items I had just bought. Now, when I look at something new, I'm already envisioning the process of it becoming faded, old, and torn.

This helps my mind to pause in that moment, so as not to be carried away by the wanting or the desire for the novelty of that object. I may still buy it, but I also learn to take good care of it because I know one day it will be old and worn.

I also appreciate more deeply the material things I already have, that they're old because they've been there for me all this time, so I don't throw them out or look down on them just because I have something newer.

Little by little, awareness and these simple practices tame the mind of desire and grasping.

As much as I enjoy and cherish my monastic life, the tendency for attachment is still alive in me. In the depth of my peace and quietude, I touch an undercurrent of yearning for someone, a loving look, a hand-holding, closeness and affection. I sit quietly and breathe with these waves of yearning. Deep in my heart, I know that true love is protecting me and the people I love.

True love lies in helping each other realize our aspirations and cultivate happiness and freedom. This requires more self-discipline and dignity than reflexively grasping something that we like or running away from something that we don't like.

In a relationship, you may start to take each other for granted like an old pair of shoes or a worn-out shirt. Then when something novel and exciting comes along, you grab it and kick the old shoes aside. New things and new people will only be new for a while. Just like a shirt or a pair of shoes, they will soon be faded and worn out, probably even sooner than expected, especially when we merely surf on their novelty and don't invest our care in them. But to remember and cherish our old love, and the many trials and tribulations we've gone through together all these years, is to be rooted in Right View and Right Thinking.

Chapter Five

REVERENCE AND RESPECT

Reverence is the nature of my love.
    —From a calligraphy by Thich Nhat Hanh

When we realize that we're the product of all of our ancestors, human and non-human, that have come before us, we see that nothing about us is uniquely our own; everything has been transmitted to us, and we feel deep reverence for all life, including ourselves, and we wish to protect ourselves and our ancestors. We practice reverence in our mindful thoughts, speech, and actions.

Often I would see retreatants bowing deeply and solemnly as they enter or exit the meditation hall, and before they sit down on a cushion or a chair in the dining hall. Children would stand quietly to look at a flower on the sidewalk and teenagers would sit contentedly underneath a tree. A young man shared in a Dharma sharing, "I was passing a tree today. I looked at it for a while, and for the first time I realized that this tree gives me life and comfort. So I sat down in its shade for a while." When the mind is free from the replay of incessant thoughts and perceptions, we're fully present for what is—a flower, a tree, a sunset, a space, a person—and we touch the immensity of it and we become in awe of it. In profound reverence, the thought of a separate self is also removed. The one who bows and the one who is bowed to become one and limitless. The truth of interbeing is fully experienced in thoughts, speech, and bodily actions.

MOTHER EARTH

Mother Earth is the great mother for all of us. She gives us birth, provides all of our basic needs, and she is there for us during our whole life and afterward. Taking refuge in Mother Earth and preserving her is nurturing and healing ourselves.

When I walk, I do my best to be in touch with Mother Earth and to receive her strength and tenderness. During many years of my life, I felt that my biological mother deserted me and abandoned me. She was violent to me verbally and physically, so it was difficult to feel nurtured by her. With the practice of returning to my roots, I have learned to be empathetic and grateful to my biological mother, and I have also discovered Mother Earth, who is also the mother of my mother. I have discovered how loving and inclusive Mother Earth is, and this daily awareness and nourishment helps heal me and my biological mother inside of me.

As monastic practitioners, we show our gratitude and reverence to Mother Earth in our way of walking gently and mindfully everywhere we go. We are also careful with the way we use Mother Earth's resources. For example, we turn on the water slowly so that the stream of water doesn't come out too forcefully and wastefully. Sisters use a cup to collect enough water to brush their teeth and wash their faces. Instead of letting water run freely from the showerhead, many of us collect water in a bucket and take a shower from it. We turn off all the lights before we leave a room. We reuse and recycle paper and plastic bottles. We compost leftover food. These small acts of gratitude and reverence nourish us and our Mind of Love.

FRACTAL IN A DOGWOOD TREE

Please join me for a short meditation exercise: let us examine a dogwood tree. You can visualize that its trunk divides into two large branches. Each of these large branches divides into smaller branches, and those smaller branches then divide into even smaller branches. This process of division repeats numerous times until it reaches the distant tips of the branches, where there are dogwood flowers.

Biologists call this phenomenon "fractal," which means repeating patterns. When you first look at a tree, it may seem complicated and random. Upon closer examination, you will discover that it has a repeating pattern throughout, from the trunk to the distant tips of its smallest branches.

Imagine yourself as a flower of this dogwood tree. You ask yourself, where am I from? How did I arrive here? Where did I obtain all of my physical and mental characteristics? Where do my personality, my joy and suffering, talents and habit energies come from?

You may tell yourself, "That's just me alone. I am unique like that." Many of us, children and adults, feel quite lost, lonely, and separated from the rest of humanity when we stand all the way out at the distant tip of the branch. Standing out there as one beautiful flower, you may feel that you are more special and beautiful than those dry, old branches underneath. You may see yourself as different and disconnected from the rest of the tree.

However, if you look deeply, you will see that you're not actually hanging out there alone in midair. Something is holding you up. You are connected to a small branch, which is connected to a bigger branch, which is connected to an even bigger branch, and this connection continues until it reaches down to the trunk of the tree. You are actually part of a fractal.

Moreover, at ground level, the tree trunk begins to spread out its roots, and interestingly enough, these roots also have a fractal repeating pattern like the tree branches. However wide and tall the tree may be, its roots will be just as wide and deep, and so there's a mirror image of the tree underneath the earth.

It's a wonderful meditation to see yourself as a tree. You can go to a tree and stand in front of it. Sometimes you may see yourself as a small plant or flower. Sometimes you may see yourself as an ancient, gigantic tree. However young or old you are, talented or not so talented, if you look deeply you will realize that you're not just a flower hanging in midair, but you are a part of a great whole. You will see that you are immense and deeply connected to life. You will feel more stable and solid. You will not be so caught by a feeling of pride or of shame. My mother went to school for only three years, but I went to school for twenty-four years. Does that make me better than my mother?

If we are more talented and endowed with more advantageous conditions than our parents, and we cut off ourselves from them, then it isn't unlike plucking a flower off its branch. The flower will not survive alone very well. However, if we stay connected to our ancestors throughout our lives, we feel solid and supported, and we can continue to discover more about ourselves.

Besides visualizing ourselves as a tree, we can also practice "tree hugging meditation." Stand in front of a tree, look at it, and breathe mindfully. When you close your eyes, you will see the image of the tree in your mind's eye. You see yourself as the tree, and then you bow to the tree, hug it, and breathe with it. In moments of stillness, you will see yourself as one with the tree. The tree is breathing, you are breathing, and there is just breath. That sense of oneness and spaciousness can heal you deeply.

ANCESTORS

Just as a tree has many roots, we too have many roots. Our roots are our ancestors—those who have come before us. First are our blood ancestors, including our parents as our youngest ancestors, then our grandparents, great-grandparents, and so on.

In addition to our blood ancestors, adoptive parents, or guardians, we also have spiritual ancestors. We are human beings, and we are also spiritual beings, and that's why we are not content to stay only at home with our family members and the material comforts there. We have a desire to reach out, to go to the mountains and the rivers, to go to practice centers and to teachers, because in us there are spiritual ancestors who always want to fully realize themselves in us.

Through evolution, we also have animal ancestors, plant ancestors, and mineral ancestors, such as rocks. Have you ever thought of yourself as having these many ancestors? How does it make you feel? Yes, you may feel ancient, like the stars themselves.

When you realize that you are so deeply connected to all of these innumerable ancestors and to life itself, you can't help but have a deep sense of reverence for yourself, for all of these ancestors and for life. How can you take care of yourself in order to show that profound reverence? How can a flower take care of itself? How does it show reverence for the rest?

In a practice center, we learn to express our reverence by the way we sit and walk with mindfulness and solidity. Every bodily action can be an expression of deep love and respect when it's done with attentiveness and care. When we perform any skills, we can also remember with gratitude that our ancestors have transmitted them to us, and now we're continuing these skills and refining them further. We don't really create or invent anything out of nothing; all capacities, talents, skills, new ideas, and inventions have their roots in previous ancestors and generations.

Protecting people, animals, plants, and minerals is another way to show reverence for life, knowing that we are intricately connected to them, and that their safety and survival are our own safety and survival. When we realize that we are all each other's ancestors, that all life, all that exists, is our ancestor, then however young we may be, we will learn to respect life and everything that is life, through the way we sit, walk, speak, and behave. We want our actions to be as beautiful as possible so that our ancestors themselves can continue beautifully.

PROTECTING ANCESTORS IN US

We practice to protect and show reverence for our ancestors by protecting ourselves. When we think of thoughts like "I am nobody," "I am not good at anything," "My father loves my sister more than he loves me," "My mother doesn't care about me," etc., they bring sadness and lethargy to our body and to our spirit, which isn't healthy for the ancestors inside us. These feelings of dejection and isolation don't reflect the truth about our nature of interbeing and interconnectedness. They make us weak and sick, unable to blossom as beautifully as we can.

Therefore, we learn to protect our thoughts about ourselves, our family members, and others. We choose to think positively, with joy and gratitude, finding ways to bring more happiness to ourselves and others.

We can also protect ourselves with our speech, speaking kind and loving words to our beloved such as, "Mom, Dad, thank you for giving me life." Our parents are ordinary people, but they perform magic by giving us life. Science can be sophisticated and advanced, but scientific technologies can't give us life and nurture us the way our parents have done all of these years.

"Thank you for being there for me. Thank you for taking this adventure with me," we tell our parents and our partners as often as we can. This is also a way to give them energy so that they can continue to be there with us, because we know we can be demanding, and being with us and taking care of us require stamina and effort.

Carrying out kind and loving bodily actions is another way to protect and show reverence to ourselves and our ancestors. Sometimes we aren't kind and loving in our thoughts, speech, and bodily actions. Sometimes others are unskillful toward us. When this happens, remember to breathe, to smile, to do sitting meditation and walking meditation to release all of the toxins, so that you don't bring those toxins into your body and mind.

CORDIAL AS NEW FRIENDS

In the Vietnamese tradition, we're taught that husbands and wives should respect one another as if we were acquaintances or new friends. In all relationships whether it's between lovers, between parents, between parents and children or between friends, we should respect each other as if we were new to each other. You wouldn't dare to say something harsh, impolite, or to do something rude or unkind to a stranger. You would want to be careful. Living together over time, it's particularly important to remain mindful of our speech and behaviors in order to protect our love and respect for one another.

In our monastic life, we have mindful manners and precepts that help us to preserve this respect. For example, before one sister offers a massage to another sister who is sick and in need of care, we join our palms into a lotus and say, "Please allow me" or "Please give me the permission to massage you." The sister would also sit up beautifully and bow back and give her permission and gratitude to us. While we're massaging our sister's body, we follow our breathing diligently. We acknowledge that this body is the body of the Buddha, the body of the Sangha and we are helping to take care of this body so that our sister can be well and continue to realize her Buddha nature and to serve the Sangha and the world. When I was very sick with Lyme disease, some of my sisters would take turns to give me a massage. One sister would recite silently the Discourse on Love during the whole time of the massage to help her mind stay peaceful, calm, and truly present. We don't usually talk while we're giving or receiving a massage so that our energy is peaceful and calm, and it also prevents our mind from wandering elsewhere, which would be a sign of disrespect. When we aren't mindful, the way we touch can be from a wrong source of energy, which can water the seed of desire or a seed of attachment in us.

In the Vietnamese tradition as well as in the monastic tradition, we don't remove our clothes in front of each other. We don't casually or blatantly expose our naked body in front of each other. This is to show dignity in our own body and respect toward ourselves. And when we're able to do that for ourselves, we can offer dignity and respect toward another person's body. This can be a wonderful practice for couples. When you touch each other's bodies, you may choose to practice mindfulness to maintain your full presence and respect. When you touch somebody carelessly, unmindfully, or disrespectfully, even if that is your brother, sister, husband, wife or children, you may injure that person, physically or psychologically. It's from this lack of attention or respect to thoughts, speech, and bodily actions that sexual abuse has taken place within the married relationship and in situations such as incest, molestation, or rape. Our careless thoughts and actions can cause great harm, both physically and psychologically, to those we love.

Unaware of our consumption, we may water the unwholesome seeds in our own mind daily through television programs, music, and food. We may say to each other things that are perverse, provocative, or unmindful. The way we've been trained to think about sex and the way we approach another person's body can feed the seeds of sexual desire, violence, and recklessness in us. Before we know it, we might impose our desire on somebody and hurt that person, not only in that moment but for life.

When a person is forced, it isn't only the physical pain that the person suffers from, but it's the unwholesome energy, the negative intention, the violence, the uncontrollable desire, the manipulation of the perpetrator that will imprint itself in every cell of the victim. Even though the body heals and the cells slough off and regenerate, the person is forever wounded because these unwholesome energies remain engraved in the consciousness of every cell.

About three years ago, I became aware that every time I'd try to recall an image of a man, my uncle's face would appear in my mind! This phenomenon had probably been taking place for many years, but I was simply unaware of it. Even when I try to visualize John or someone else I love and respect, I cannot hold his image for more than a split second before my uncle's face will appear and replace it. This image of my uncle is so overpowering that my mind is literally not able to visualize the face of another man as it really is. There are only two exceptions to this: When

I try to visualize my blood brother, Sonny, or Thay, then I can see them clearly in my mind. Even then, if I try to hold their image for a while, it still turns into the face of my uncle. Since I was nine years old, I always tried to avoid looking at my uncle or being around him, but evidently it was not possible to delete his existence from my mind. His face has lived on in my store consciousness.

A traumatic experience can leave a deep imprint in our mind that affects us in the most subtle ways. Some people may block the experience out of their mind consciousness in order to protect their sanity, but then it becomes a habit to leave the body and to be oblivious to the present moment. Haunted by violent and perverse images, sounds, and sensations, some victims of sexual abuse actually become perpetrators. Thus, it is crucial that we are aware of the different coping mechanisms that we might have used to adapt as children. We learn to mindfully send positive messages to our body and mind, protecting our six senses and bringing in only healthy inputs, as reflected in the Fifth Mindfulness Training about mindful consumption. When negative or haunting thoughts arise, we need to acknowledge them right away, breathe, relax, and release them. We may say to ourselves, "I am here," or "Thank you for healing. Thank you for being whole. I love you so."

PURITY AS A PROCESS

Two years into my monastic life, one day I came to the hermitage with some sisters to visit Thay. Thay asked me to come into the library. Then he sat down and started talking to me. At first, I wasn't sure where Thay was heading with his talk, but then I realized that he was teaching me about sex and sexuality. I felt like a teenager, and Thay was my father trying his best to talk about an uncomfortable subject. I was quite embarrassed and confused, because I was already thirty-two years old. Then Thay came to a conclusion, "My child, the experiences that you have gone through in your life may make it more difficult for you. But if you know how to practice, these experiences can teach you a lot, and you can help many people. Purity does not mean that you have not gone through any experiences. Purity is a process of purification."

Thay's teaching that "Purity is a process of purification" has helped me not to have any complex toward myself, my body, or my life. I have learned to purify my own thoughts about my past sexual experiences as well as about my present sexual energy with the Right View of interbeing. I have also learned to purify the way I speak to myself and the way I behave toward my body and mind. Through this process of purification of my thoughts, speech, and bodily actions, I touch purity, and I don't have a complex of inferiority, superiority, or equality in this matter whatsoever. Most of us have experienced abuse, whether we are women or men, and whether it's sexual abuse, verbal abuse, or mental abuse. We may hold these complexes and discrimination toward ourselves. However, if we learn to purify our three karmas of thoughts, bodily actions, and speech, we touch purity, and this is the purest form of purity.

STORY OF KIEU AND PURITY

In 2003, I wrote a letter to Thay and shared with him that, "Thay, I see myself as the Kieu of the twenty-first century having gone through so many trials and tribulations." This is in reference to an epic poem about a young woman named Kieu, written by the famous Vietnamese poet Nguyen Du in the nineteenth century. Kieu came from an upstanding family, and she fell in love with a young man while she was going on a trip with her younger sister and brother. This young man was also well educated and sincere. They felt an instant deep connection as soon as they saw each other. They were able to see each other again only one more time, and they made the vow that they would become husband and wife for the rest of their lives. Soon after that, a great misfortune happened to her family, when her father was falsely accused of receiving bribery. The officials had been bribed, and they took this accusation as something true in order to take advantage of the situation. They ransacked his house, took away all his possessions, put him in prison, and made the family pay money in order to bail him out of prison. He was an elderly man, and his daughter Kieu didn't think her father could endure this hardship in prison. Out of deep love and gratitude for her father, she agreed to be in an arranged marriage in order to receive the dowry of the exact amount of money that was needed to bail out her father. Unfortunately, this arranged marriage was also a trick; a woman set this up so she could buy innocent girls to be prostitutes for her. As a result, Kieu was sold into a house of prostitutes.

For fifteen years she was sold from one house to another. Occasionally, she met some men who loved her, but then they either betrayed her or they could not protect her entirely. For fifteen years she went through trials and tribulations. In the end, she jumped into a river to commit suicide, but she was saved and able to return to her family. The young man Kieu loved had married her younger sister. When Kieu returned, he wanted to marry her in order to connect their love again. She said to him in response to his request, "This purity I want to keep. It is the only way. Please help me to keep this purity."

I was deeply moved when I read this line. This person was a prostitute for fifteen years. Her body was exchanged for money, and she talked about purity. What is her purity? Her purity was her dignity in herself, regardless of her circumstance. Her purity was her love for this young man, constant all these years. All she asked him was, "Please allow me to become a nun. If you don't allow me to be a nun, my parents don't allow me to be a nun, and you want all of us to live in the same house together as a family, then please allow me to keep my body pure. Allow me to be your friend instead of your sexual partner. Sex will not bring more intimacy, because my body has gone through too much already. I'm tired and weary of it. Only our friendship can help us to continue our love and reverence for one another. My love has always been pure. If you help me to hold our relationship in this way, then my body is pure."

This is a radical way to look at purity, especially in the nineteenth century in Vietnam. Purity is often equated with virginity, but more profoundly, purity is the way we hold reverence and commitment for the dignity of our body and mind. In modern times, many people don't value the importance of virginity. We might even see sex as bait for entertainment and consumerism. Sex doesn't have to mean anything, and it doesn't have to matter. But the truth is that every experience is deposited in our store consciousness. When we go through a sexual experience without reverence, without love, without recognizing the interbeing nature between suffering and happiness, then we're abusing our own body and the other person's body. We prevent ourselves from ever experiencing true happiness. Only when we learn to cherish and protect our body and mind can we find someone with the same values, and we can care for each other in the spirit of these six elements of true love. Then our love can be mutual and respectful.

REVERENCE IN GIFT GIVING

The way you offer gifts can also show reverence. In the Vietnamese tradition, we always present an object to someone with our two hands. It is not the monetary value of the gift, but it is our true presence and recognition of that person that makes the gift priceless. If the giver is fully present, and the receiver is also truly present, then the gift is long-lasting in our memory. Once I was given a cough drop, and I received it solemnly with two hands. It stayed in my pocket for three winter months. Each time I touched it, I smiled, remembering how it was given and received with pure love and joy.

UGLY APPLE TREE

While I was severely sick, I felt waves of despair every so often. One morning, the wave was so strong that I just wanted to check out and vanish. Even so, I made the effort to walk to the dining hall for breakfast. I was walking ever so slowly, investing mindfulness in every step just to be able to hold that deep despair in me. As I was walking away from the nunnery, I saw an apple tree that I had seen many times before. That morning, it appeared as the ugliest tree I had ever seen in my life. It was so dry, barren, and perversely naked. The trunk was contorted, and the branches were like gross arthritic knuckles. It was horrible looking, and it was exactly how I was feeling about myself at that moment in body and spirit. I was that tree right there in that moment.

Then my right thinking reminded me that only three months before, when Thay was there in November, that tree had many leaves and a lot of fruit. The apples weren't perfectly round, but they were sweet, and the children were all over that tree, tugging on the fruit with long sticks. The tree had been full of life and gifts then. With that thought, something in me was soothed. Sometimes you go through life and you feel so helpless, ashamed, deserted, or barren like that tree and you want to escape from all of it, and being in nature can save your life. Nature can help remind you of the wisdom inside you. The force of life is always present, and all of our ancestors are there, holding us and supporting us to go through it, if only we can touch that awareness and not pluck ourselves from this life force, like plucking a flower off a branch. In one moment, life didn't mean anything to me, and in the next moment, I could see myself in the apple tree and say to it, "You are okay, and I am also okay." I was able to smile and continue the walk to the dining hall.

That apple tree right now is full of flowers, and it will soon bear fruit again. If you look closely, many of the leaves have holes and distorted brown edges from some kind of infection. Still, it does its best to take care of itself, and its roots, leaves, flowers, and fruits are its continuations. We, too, as both spiritual and human beings, can always do our best to show our reverence to the gifts that we've received, to whatever it is that we've been given.

We possess more gifts than we can ever fathom. Our parents are ordinary people. They make mistakes. They may be full of mistakes that can wound us deeply. Still, we can show them our gratitude and reverence because they have given us the gift of life. However vast the ocean is, it is still only a part of life. Yet our parents have given us the gift of life itself, and we can take care of this great gift for ourselves and for our ancestors.

Generations of our spiritual ancestors have also built bridges and opened the path for us. Each time I touch the earth, I visualize a sea of monastic ancestors in sanghati robes, and I feel that I, too, can follow their examples and overcome my obstacles. This is the process of purification, purifying the wounds and pain that we carry in our body and in our mind. Even if you feel that your leaves are burnt and distorted, your fruit not full, red, juicy, and delicious, if you take each step in awareness, in peace, and in reverence, you can touch the beauty in yourself and in life. In that moment, there is no inferiority or superiority complex whatsoever. You can begin anew every such moment.

As human beings, we are a part of a repeating pattern, of a fractal, and we are repeating our ancestors both positively in terms of their talents and virtues, and negatively in terms of their illnesses, sufferings, and habit energies. Nevertheless, we're never stuck there like a flower on the tip of a branch. We can purify and renew ourselves and our ancestors in the most beautiful ways. With each step in gratitude and in Noble Silence, we touch beauty, wholesomeness, and truth. Purity is a process of purification, and it is a daily practice.

MANY MOTHERS

My mother disappeared when I was twelve years old. Even when she was still alive, I hardly had any time with her. I didn't live with her until I was six years old, and during the six years that I did live with her, she was outside the house working most of the day. At one point, I calculated that I actually had less than a few months with my mother in my entire life.

In my monastic life, I have learned to discover my mother deeply. Genetically, she is in every cell of my body with her twenty-three chromosomes. Even though you may have never met my mother, you can see my mother's features through me. Perhaps I smile more often than my mother, so that is one kind thing I am doing for her. These days, I don't cry as much as my mother used to, and I breathe and smile while I am crying, so I don't suffer that much even at those times. That is another kind action I do for my mother.

I also have many other mothers. Living in a monastic community, my older and younger monastic brothers and sisters are also my mothers. Their manual labor, their practice, and their loving acceptance provide me a home in which I can rest and heal. A wounded or sick animal searches for a quiet and safe place to lie down, rest, and heal. When I first came to Blue Cliff Monastery, I was that wounded animal. My body and mind were in such deep pain and exhaustion that I literally just wanted to lie down and sleep for three months. I had to find a place where I could feel safe to do so.

My elder sister, Sister The Nghiem, also known as Sister True Vow, came to talk to me. She told me, "Sister Dang Nghiem, please stay here with us. I have done my best to help build this community in such a way that sisters can feel comfortable to rest and to take care of their illness. Please give Blue Cliff a chance."

I will always remember the statement Sister True Vow made, "Please give Blue Cliff a chance." It really meant, please give yourself a chance. I did give myself a chance. I stayed. My sisters provided me a safe and accepting place so I could sleep all I needed to. I still sleep a lot. At least once or twice a week, I sleep all day or half a day because I feel exhausted or there is too much pain to bear. Many mornings after sitting meditation, I go back to sleep until breakfast or even through breakfast. I have jokingly told my sisters—with mixed feelings of awe and sadness—that I am sleeping half of my life, making up for all the sleep deprivation while I was in school for twenty-four years. I even find myself looking forward to sleep more than to sitting meditation at times.

HEALING IN DREAMS

I console myself that I am also practicing during sleep. During my wakeful hours, I do my best to cultivate mindfulness in my thoughts, speech, and bodily actions, and this energy of awareness penetrates into my sleep. Before, when I dreamed, I was often a victim, finding myself in dire situations and reacting to them. When the day is spent in chaos and forgetfulness, dreams can become festered with psychological wounds, reinforcing and perpetuating them further. With awareness, I can actually hear myself thinking through the process and see myself making choices. In my dream, I can actually know what is going on, and I can make a choice to do something or not to do something.

This is transformation and healing at the base. Mindfulness can be there to work with your store consciousness while you're resting and sleeping. The presence and the practice of my monastic brothers and sisters allow me the opportunity to practice and to heal. I hope that you also provide a safe and supportive environment for yourself, your partners and children, so that you can lie down, rest and sleep when you feel tired, sick, or wounded.

Sometimes we judge ourselves and one another, "Why did you lose your job? How long will you be out of work? You're not performing your duty and responsibility. You're not worthy." This kind of judgment and criticism only deepens the malady within us, both physically and spiritually.

On the other hand, an attitude of reverence gives each person time and space, trusting one another's best intentions. "Trust me that I am doing my best to take care of myself, and thus of you. I also trust that you are doing your best to take care of yourself, and thus of me, and I will do my best to support you in this endeavor."

Sometimes as parents, we think we know what is best for our children. With the best of intentions, we drive them to do what we want, because we believe that what is best for us should be best for them. The mystic Khalil Gibran said, "Your children are not your children. They are the sons and daughters of life, longing for itself." In reverence, we offer respect and trust to the ideals and aspirations that we each have, even our children, and the choices that they may make.

In our partnership, we also have a tendency to force what we want on each other. Even in our community, we also have strong ideas and views, and we push them on each other.

However, in the practice of reverence we see that the other person is deeply connected to us. We also trust the spiritual ancestors in them, providing them wisdom and guidance. They have ideals and aspirations in them that we wouldn't want to impede.

To me, this is true love. Sometimes when we love someone, we want to hold onto that person. Not only do we want them to conform to our ideas and views, but we also want to hold onto them physically. Then, when they're right there next to us, we take them for granted. To be able to respect our beloved's time and space, to encourage them to explore their aspirations, to be free to live as fully as possible, even if it means we have to be apart from them—this is the deepest form of reverence.

Journal Entry—Email to My Brother Sonny

December 1, 2013

Yes, precious love, I miss you and Sunee, too, a lot a lot! Can't believe still that she has manifested in our lives and made such a big difference in our lives. Every time I look at her photos by my bed, I smile and want to cry at the same time.

Em oi [Dear younger brother], it looks like I also begin to have the onset of diabetes, too. I've been checking up on HgA1C, a very specific marker for diabetes since I got Lyme disease. This last blood test two weeks ago showed that it's HIGH. I've been feeling deeply sad for the last four days. I just sat in meditation and then tears just streamed down my face. I got neurological Lyme as a chronic illness, and now I've got another chronic illness! The news just took the wind out of me!

Then two nights ago, I had a dream. I was hungry, and I went in a restaurant with a few people. I went upstairs to use the restroom. What I saw was a gigantic room, all made of green marble, from the ceiling, to the walls, to the floor. It was incredibly imposing and magnificent. I kept looking for the restroom, then I saw there were squatting toilets right out there by the wall! There were some doors, too, but I used the squatting one because it was right there. When I stood up and walked back, I realized that urine was seeping through the floor. That huge room was used as the restroom! I saw a group of visitors from afar, all dressed up formally. A big group of people in suits was also cleaning the space with mops and other implements. I thought to myself: Ah, this building is historic and precious, so people want to preserve it as it is. The toilet system is outdated, but they could not renovate it because then they would have to change the building. . . .

In meditation, I brought up the dream. I had no idea what it meant. Then slowly it came to me that the incredibly ancient, imposing, and magnificent room is my body, which has been transmitted to me by our mother and grandmother and ancestors. Yes, it has a faulty toilet system, but it is nonetheless precious. It is worthy of preserving and taking care of. The many people working to maintain the place are the buddhas, bodhisatvas, people, animals, plants, and minerals that help uphold and sustain my life all of these years and the rest of my years. I cannot just want to throw it all away, just because I have a fearful vision that my old age will be full of sickness and pain.

I saw I've inherited the joint pain from our mother and grandmother, and now the diabetes from her and from her ancestors.

I've inherited from our mother this body and mind, with many strengths and beauties, but also with many shortcomings and sicknesses. I cannot choose some and reject others. Our mother has passed away a long time ago, but she is so alive in my body and in your body. What we can do is to do our best to take care of our health, so that she has a chance to heal and transform and to live a life of peace and joy in us.

This dream really helped me to see a greater picture of my life and to exit my deep sadness and despair. Well, I still get teary easily, but I can also recognize the many many good conditions available to me in the present moment. I continue to eat a healthy diet, and I will make a point not to eat candy or many sweets from now on (I did have the sweet soup *che troi nuoc* last night, and it was yummy). I continue to exercise every day. I am in really good shape, honey. My abdomen is flat and strong. I have a bit of joint pain and muscle pain, because Lyme always gets worse when the weather is cold. But I still smile, because I know I am doing the best I can to take care of my body for myself, for our mother and ancestors, for you and Sunee.

Em oi, please also take good care of yourself. Be more committed to taking better care of your health with concrete steps (and you know what they are). Have more discipline, precious love. Sunee depends on you. She needs you to be healthy and happy, so that she can be healthy and happy. You've transmitted to her your body and the body of our ancestors. You continue to transmit to her through your daily actions and choices. Please make them wisely and lovingly.

I love you sincerely,

Your beloved sister and Sunee's number one fan

CHOOSING EACH DAY

While Thay was cutting a strand of my hair as a part of my monastic ordination, he was also reading this poem line by line, "Shaving my head completely today, I vow to transform my afflictions and to help all living beings."

Tears streamed down my face as I repeated these lines after him. Then he bestowed on me three ceremonial robes and read another gatha for me to repeat, "How beautiful is the sanghati robe of a nun. It is a field of merits. I vow to wear it life after life after life."

Thus, I made the great vow on the day I shaved my head. However, that wasn't the only time I made that vow. I choose to be a nun each day. It's just as when you get married. You make a vow to be with a person for the rest of your life, but unfortunately, if you make that vow only once and then forget about it, the marriage will not succeed.

I am still young. I am a nun, but I am also too human. There are still tendencies in me to become attached to another person. Mindful manners and mindfulness practices are ways for me to be with myself and to transform my suffering while cultivating positive seeds in myself. This is true freedom and true love. Holding onto somebody will bring suffering to me and to that person. Our love may turn into disappointment, disillusionment, resentment, and hate.

I make a daily choice to be a monastic practitioner, and this infuses me with energy. I don't feel obligated by my vows or that I am burdened by them.

When you know that you have a choice to be in a relationship or not, whether it's in a marriage or in a community, you take the initiative to care for that relationship.

When I learn to cherish my own space, time, and freedom, then I also respect and cherish the space, time, and freedom of the other person. When we lack spaciousness inside, we become needy, and we put demands on the other person to entertain us, to fulfill our life for us. If the person isn't able to perform these tasks, we complain, blame and feel saddened or disappointed.

Once we're able to cultivate space, time, and freedom in ourselves, we would never want to take those things away from, or put demands on the other person. Loving each other with this spaciousness in both of us, we come together, not out of neediness or expectation, but because we're spacious and we can harmonize our space together. We have much to offer to each other and we don't have to claim, grasp, or hold onto anything. The union of people who have space and freedom within themselves can bring profound joy, happiness, and discovery. This is true for all people, monastic and lay.

When we feel inspired, we may speak eloquent and passionate words to our beloved, but these may be words with wings, vanishing in time.

In true love, there must be recognition, respect, and support for each other's aspirations, ideals, and endeavors. If your loved ones have a vision about a project or they're working on something meaningful to them, you can be truly present, listen and help them realize their projects, and rejoice in their achievements. You can only do this when you are able to offer yourself the same respect and support, and this comes from a place of spaciousness within yourself. You and your beloved also learn to respect each other's space, time, and freedom. It's like a garden that's beautiful and healthy because the flowers and the trees have sufficient conditions to be themselves and to thrive.

LOVE IS EVERY MOMENT

True love is not something idealistic or far-fetched; it's realized in every moment. When you love someone, do you wish for your beloved to be truly happy? Whatever it takes for your beloved to be happy, can you wish that for him regardless of yourself?

That is true love. You wish that person to be free, to be happy, to enjoy wherever he or she is, instead of feeling self-pity and asking, "Why is he not with me? Why is she not paying attention to me? How can that person be so joyful without me?"

When thinking about the other person, if you feel tension and constriction in your body, in your feeling and in your thinking, you know it isn't true love in that moment.

True love can manifest in the moment you sit quietly and return to your own breathing, instead of going toward your beloved and trying to get his or her attention. True love is in the moment you allow the beloved to be in peace, rejoicing in his or her space and time alone and with other people.

You also learn to practice true love for yourself, enjoying your own space and time, comfortable in your own company and in the company of whoever you are with. You nourish the beautiful qualities of your beloved in yourself and diligently transform your suffering and limitations. Thus, you neither feel separated when apart nor estranged when you are together. This is the practice of reverence for oneself and reverence for another person, and this is also the insight of interbeing.

Chapter Six

HEALING

May I choose this breath to be my home.
May I choose this step to be my home.
May I choose this smile to be my home.
May I accept this Earth to be my home.

This breath is my home.
This step is my home.
This smile is my home.
This Earth is my home.

There is only home.
There is only home.
Home.
Home.

Another element of true love is karuna. In Sanskrit, karuna is the capacity to relieve and transform suffering and sorrows. It's about the removal of suffering, both in oneself and in another person.

Karuna has been translated in the past as compassion. However, the word compassion implies "a feeling of wanting to help someone." Thus, compassion does not effectively convey the capacity to relieve and remove suffering as is implied in karuna.

The root words of "compassion" are also problematic since "com" is a prefix that means "together," and "passion" is defined in Webster's Dictionary as "a strong feeling of enthusiasm or excitement, a strong feeling (such as anger) that causes you to act in a dangerous way, a very strong dislike, a strong sexual or romantic feeling for someone, or something that you enjoy or love doing very much."

Because these forms of passion can be either positive, or negative, unwholesome and destructive—such as excessive passion for sex, power, or fame—the word "compassion" can be misleading as a translation of karuna.

Moreover, "compassion" might also be understood as "suffering together," which would also be an inaccurate interpretation of karuna. For example, a doctor does not need to suffer along with his or her patients. A doctor only needs to be skilled enough to make an accurate diagnosis and offer an effective treatment plan to help relieve the patient from the symptoms and the illness itself.

The Buddhist insight reveals that when ignorance dissipates, clarity arises. It's like saying that when darkness is removed, light manifests.

Similarly, when suffering is removed, healing becomes present.

In this spirit, we can attempt to translate karuna as "the capacity to heal" or "healing." The word healing is direct and straightforward for people to understand: there's an ailment and there's a process of transformation that takes place. To heal is to become healthy and well again.

In true love, there must be healing. The healer, the healed, and the healing process inter-are. In the practice of true love, we must be able to exercise the capacity to heal ourselves first, so that we may offer it to the one we love—whether that is a single person, a group of people, a nation, or the world.

With the practice of mindfulness, healing can take place through different pathways. For example, when we're sick, we have an opportunity to practice deeply and to heal from that illness, not only physically but also psychologically and spiritually. Healing can also take place through mindfulness of the abuses and traumas that we've been through, in the relationships we have with ourselves and with others, and in our views about birth and death. These are important areas that we can explore under the theme of karuna.

HEALING IN ILLNESS

I was trained as a medical doctor. However, it has not been my medical knowledge but the practice of mindfulness that has helped me to listen to my body and to take care of myself more effectively over the past fifteen years as a nun. I have learned that there is an art of being sick, which enables us to take care of our illness with dignity, empathy, and joy so that transformation and healing may take place in every moment.

MASTERPIECE OF THE TICK

In our monastic life, each year at the end of the Winter Retreat we have a practice called Shining Light where we give feedback to each other about our strengths and areas to improve.

When it was my turn to receive the shining light, one sister said to me, "Dear elder sister, I know you have a lot of physical pain, but I am so grateful to you because when you join the Sangha activities you are always joyful and fresh and loving, and you leave the pain behind in your room. I am very grateful to you."

Another sister said to me, "You are a masterpiece of the tick and compassion." She had just learned the word "masterpiece" in English a few days before, and she used it in my shining light. Of all the titles, diplomas, and degrees I have received, I must admit that I delight most in this title that my sister offered me, "Masterpiece of the Tick."

The truth is that it takes a lot for a person to accept that he or she is sick and that there is a need for a pause in order to take care of the body. In our society we're trained to be busy; busyness reflects a person's value and worth. We run on adrenaline. We run like a car on empty, until we completely break down.

When we have physical pain or psychological discomfort, we may not hear it at all until it's severe because our mind is preoccupied and full of noise, as though we're in an open market, where we cannot hear a soft cry or a fallen object.

Even when we recognize that there's something wrong with our body or mind, we turn to entertainment and recreational activities to divert our attention from the pain, or we take medication to mask the pain, instead of stopping our busyness in order to come back to ourselves and take care of the root of our problem.

THE ART OF BEING SICK

In April 2006, after six months of being in our newly established Bat Nha Monastery in Vietnam, I returned to Deer Park Monastery. I felt extremely tired and weak. I would try to attend Sangha activities, but I would come back to my room feeling exhausted. At first I thought it would pass after a few weeks, but it continued on for months.

We doctors are known for not going to see other doctors when we're sick. Many of us try to handle things ourselves, and that was my case. I tried to exercise, eat more, rest more, and to keep making efforts to attend Sangha functions. My symptoms of fatigue, lethargy, dizziness, and forgetfulness became worse—and finally—I went to see a doctor.

Just by taking my vital signs, they discovered that my blood pressure was only 84/59. One option was to take medication to increase my blood pressure, but that would cause many short- and long-term side effects, including fluctuating blood pressure, mood swings, and osteoporosis. I had always been resistant to taking medications, and the possible severe side effects made this option even less appealing to me.

I could have also taken Chinese herbal medicine, but at that time my faith in Chinese medicine wasn't strong. I had been healthy all my life, so

I wasn't used to being sick. Having seen sick patients during my medical training had never brought home to me the possibility that I, too, might be sick one day.

As a nun, I didn't seek entertainment or recreational activities or analgesics to suppress my symptoms, but the old habit energy in me still prevented me from stopping completely and acknowledging that I was really sick. I had never been seriously sick in my life, so I could not fathom that I could be sick now. Denial and resistance were still strong, so that I spent over three years trying to deal with my symptomatic low blood pressure without any sort of medication.

I used mindfulness to help me to cope with my symptoms. For example, I would stand up very slowly to avoid the sudden dizziness upon changing posture. I walked slowly up the hill to minimize the shortness of breath. I dwelled more deeply in the present moment, because I saw that it was truly the only moment that I had. This measure also helped reduce the forgetfulness that I was experiencing along with the low blood pressure.

I adjusted well to my illness, but it nevertheless weakened me physically and affected every aspect of my life.

Then one day Auntie Thuy Do, a long-term practitioner at Deer Park, said to me, "Dear Sister, you make a difference in the lives of many young people, and we want you to be healthy so you can continue this work. I know of this Chinese doctor who is very good, and I'm willing to drive you there to get the medicine. Please give it a chance. Don't answer me right away. I will be here at the monastery for a few days, and you can tell me of your decision later."

Something inside me at that moment was open to this option. A few hours later I told our lay friend that I was willing to go see the Chinese herbalist, and she was surprised by my sudden compliance. It took only three months for me to feel less symptomatic, and after a year or so I could see my health recovering. I continued to take the herbal medicine for two years, and I felt my energy return to what it had been before. Even though my systolic blood pressure only went up to the high nineties, and the diastolic blood pressure to the high sixties, I was no longer symptomatic. On Lazy Days, I could hike and roam the mountains with my brothers and sisters with no problem. From that experience I learned to listen to my body more closely, to accept my illness, and to seek help more promptly.

CONTRACTING NEURO-LYME DISEASE

I enjoyed good health again for almost two years. Right before the Winter Retreat 2010–11 began, I volunteered to go to the Magnolia Grove Practice Center in Mississippi where many Bat Nha brothers and sisters relocated. After the winter, I went on the Southeast Asia Teaching Tour with Thay and a group of monastic brothers and sisters. A few weeks after I came back to the United States from the tour, I began to experience excruciating headaches throughout the day. The stabbing pain would wake me up several times in the night. I also felt tired and drowsy and slept a lot during the day.

My hearing was also affected to the point that I couldn't hear the activity bell. One time a younger brother asked me, "Elder sister, why don't you stop when there's a bell?" I replied, "Was there a bell? I didn't hear anything!" So from then on, if I saw brothers and sisters stopping, I would stop with them. One time, I was at the head of the serving table and I saw a girl standing still outside the door, so I stood still and breathed... and breathed...and breathed. All the younger brothers and sisters standing behind me also stood still, because they saw me stopping. After a long while, one sister asked me politely, "Elder sister, are you hearing something?" I said, "Is that the bell?" They all replied, "No!" and we laughed.

My differential diagnoses included a severe flu, recurrent hypotension, and Lyme disease. I had learned about Lyme disease briefly in medical school, and back then, it was an extremely rare illness. It was also not prevalent in Mississippi, as on the East Coast, so even though the possibility crossed my mind, I didn't consider it seriously. I kept thinking that if I ever developed swelling and pain in my joints, then it would confirm the diagnosis of Lyme disease.

In retrospect, it's true that I had migratory joint pain, phantom-like, appearing and disappearing in different joints like a fleeting wisp of wind, varied in intensity and perceptibility. My mind was unclear and clouded at times, and so I could not recognize this phantom-like pain as migratory joint pain.

I also had the classic Lyme disease "bull's eye" lesion, on the medial (inner) side of my right knee, but I mistook it for a bruise from clearing wood in the forest.

The severe headaches and drowsiness clouded my judgment, and I thought my body was simply tired from the trip to Southeast Asia, and I was coming down with a bad flu. When I wasn't feeling feverish and drowsy, I would continue to follow Sangha activities. I also played volleyball whenever I could muster enough energy, and it gave me a chance to interact with my brothers and sisters joyfully.

In June 2011, I attended my brother's wedding in California, representing our parents to speak to his bride's parents, and served as the master of ceremony at the wedding.

On the night I came back to Magnolia Grove Monastery, my right knee felt painful. The next morning it was visibly swollen, and I was limping. I thought to myself, "Oh no, this is definitely Lyme disease!" I went to see the doctor that same day, told him about my symptoms, and said that I probably had Lyme disease. Dr. Korkern exclaimed, "I'll be darned. I think you do, too!" We both laughed. The diagnosis was made almost two months late, but it was still an improvement from my last experience with sickness. With the hypotension it took me three years to agree to take medication, and with Lyme disease, I began the antibiotic treatment on that very day.

Thay's US Tour in 2011 started in August, and I decided to follow him and the Sangha for the entire three-month tour while I was on two kinds of antibiotics, doxycycline and rocephine (IM injection), plus the antimalarial drug Plaquenil—a mixture that targeted the Lyme disease bacteria in the bloodstream, in the cells, and in the cysts. I could have opted to rest at the monastery, but I reasoned that, given Thay's age, this might be his last tour, and I sincerely wished to be able to accompany my Teacher. I also trusted that Thay's energy and the Sangha's joy would carry me through.

During the tour, I had diarrhea at least ten times a day; it was worst in the morning, and I allowed myself not to go to morning sitting meditation without feeling guilty. The diarrhea persisted for over one year, and it led to a bleeding hemorrhoid; I knew from medical school that a hemorrhoid resulted from chronic constipation, but I discovered from my own experience that chronic diarrhea also led to severe bleeding as well. Food tasted like cardboard, but I chewed slowly and mindfully.

I could not go hiking at all while we were at YMCA of the Rockies, because I had severe shortness of breath and sun sensitivity. So I went swimming indoors instead. I didn't think I could make it through the whole tour, so I just took one retreat at a time and, for the most part, just one bout of pain at a time.

I also noticed that my response was at times slow and my memory and concentration impaired. For example, in the past on a rare occasion during a Dharma talk, Thay would pause for a moment in search of a particular word or a particular name. Usually, I would be the one to prompt Thay with that piece of information because I could project my voice from a distance. Yet during the tour, I actually gave Thay the wrong information three times! Thankfully, Sister Chan Khong was there to correct it immediately. From then on, I didn't dare to offer Thay information on the spot anymore.

I was relieved when I made it to Blue Cliff Monastery, which was the last segment of our tour. In my dream one night, I saw that I was walking through a dark corridor. I was going to see someone, and my heart was full of excitement and anticipation. When I came to the spacious room, the door was slightly open. It was dark and deserted inside, but I decided to go in anyway. In a faint light I could see a bed in the corner of the room. Someone was lying there, facing the wall. All of my fluttering emotions subsided at that point, and I quietly lay down next to that person, cupping the person's body with my own and whispering, "I didn't know you were so tired!"

When I woke up from the dream, I sat still for a long time. I realized that the person lying on the bed in the dream was myself, and that I needed to stay in one place in order to take better care of my illness. Thay and some of my monastic siblings helped me to choose Blue Cliff Monastery as a place for me to rest and recover. I remember after one late-night talk at Hoa Nghiem Temple in Virginia, I went back to the room and cried silently in the dark. My teardrops felt the size of pearls. They weren't tears of sadness, but of deep joy. I felt deeply loved and understood, which gave me more energy to continue. I knew I had to entrust myself in the care of my sisters and brothers. This is the practice of letting go of sadness, fear, pride, and resistance, and of taking refuge in oneself and in others for transformation and healing to be possible.

I finished the course of antibiotics toward the end of the US Tour, and soon after, the severe headaches returned and my cognitive function seemed to become more severely impaired. I had poor concentration. I found myself having difficulty recalling a piece of information or a past event. As I tried to remember the name of a sister from Magnolia Grove Monastery, four days had passed and I still could not recall it. Finally I had to ask another sister, and she looked at me in surprise as she answered my question. I had never been very good with names, but it became obvious that I could not even recall promptly the names of the monastic sisters I was living with.

I discovered that whatever weakness we have as our baseline will become even weaker when we're sick.

I also developed speech difficulty. I was fluent in English and Vietnamese, but slowly I saw that when I tried to speak English I would mispronounce words. Because English wasn't my native language, I had trained myself to listen to my own speech and to correct myself whenever I made a mistake. Thanks to this habit, I was able to recognize that I made many more mistakes than usual. Many times a day I would mispronounce words, misuse words (consultation became consolidation), or transpose syllables (kitchen became chicken). I was one of the main translators for Thay and the Sangha for many years. Now I became nervous and uneasy when it was my turn to translate Thay's talk.

Even thoughts became repetitive, such as "I want to go go go." As these mistakes arose more frequently, the surge of frustration or despair also intensified. I came back to my breathing to calm the waves of emotion and patiently corrected myself each time. It was thanks to mindfulness that I was able to detect these symptoms early. If I hadn't had mindfulness and the habit of paying attention to my own speech, bodily actions, and thoughts, these things could have gone unnoticed.

There are patients with Neuro-Lyme disease who are totally unaware of their symptoms because they're so engrossed in their work and duties, or because they're going through other crises in their lives. When family members begin to notice their cognitive impairments or their personality changes, the disease is already quite advanced. There are cases where people park their cars in front of their house, but they don't go inside because they don't know for sure if that is really their home. It's likely that their store consciousness recognizes that it's their home, but their mind consciousness isn't stable and clear enough to know this. So they park the car in front of the house, but they just sit there for hours.

I could see where my mind was headed. I could become so forgetful. I had been practicing mindfulness diligently, so whatever arose in the moment, I was aware of, but my mind could not dwell on that object for long. For example, I was going to do something, but on the way I had forgotten what I was going to do, or what I was going to say, or what I was thinking. My mind was already racing to other thoughts or it was simply in a state of drowsiness or blurriness.

One day I wanted to work on an article and I began to write, "I am happy to be hear." I stared at the computer screen: something didn't look right. I realized that I had written "hear" instead of "here." A simple word like "exercise" would also become confusing to spell. I tried to write it five times, and it still didn't look right! Writing, which had always been dear to me, now became alienating and a struggle. It would take half an hour for me to write a short email.

I also had speech and writing difficulties in Vietnamese. These cognitive impairments were frightening to me. I had worked so hard to gain these skills and knowledge, and now they were evaporating right in front of me! Every time I discovered a new symptom, I sat quietly and breathed in order to be there for the sadness and fear that arose along with the awareness of that symptom.

I learned a lot about myself through this process, but I must admit that I wasn't always grateful for the sickness. However, my right thinking helped me to be thankful to be sick while I was still young, physically healthy, and mentally stable enough to hold it, heal it, and grow from it.

THE SECOND ARROW

The Buddha gave a wonderful teaching about "the second arrow." Imagine a person being shot with an arrow on his or her left arm. This is very painful. However, if a second arrow is shot into the same wound, the pain would not only double or triple, but it would be exponential.

When we experience a physical or mental pain, it is the first arrow. If we allow our mind to engender anger, fear, worry, despair, denial, etc., these would be the second, third, or fourth arrows that worsen our situation dramatically. Thus, when we have a physical or mental illness, we can be more aware of our own bodily reactions as well as our own feelings and perceptions.

We learn to ease fears, worries, and anxieties with the practices of deep relaxation, mindful breathing, walking meditation, and sitting meditation. Mindfulness helps prevent us from shooting the second arrow into our illness, which only worsens the situation, clouds our judgment, and takes away our energy to heal. Our body has an incredible capacity to heal. Our mind can endure any sort of pain. However, if we cloud our mind and weaken our body with denial, worries, and fears, we actually deprive ourselves of the strength we need to heal ourselves.

As I began to notice cognitive impairments in myself, I purposely tried not to read about Lyme disease. One reason for this was that I was experiencing frequent headaches. Also, I could read a whole page of a book and not understand it. After reading it again, I still didn't understand it. My reading comprehension was affected, and I didn't want to frustrate myself further.

I also felt that if I read too much about the disease, I might identify with symptoms suggested in the book, and that could cause me more anxiety.

Sister Bamboo was my roommate, and she did everything she could to help take care of me. She checked out some books on Lyme disease, so she could understand it and help me. I was grateful for her efforts, but I told her that on my part, I would learn from my own body and tell her what symptoms I was developing.

Up to this point, after having discontinued the antibiotics, I was taking only herbal medicine from a kind Vietnamese herbalist in Vermont, Dr. Quang, who had made the commitment to treat our monastic brothers and sisters for free whenever we came to him.

The course of my illness took a turn when Judy Myerson, one of our long-term practitioners, overheard that I had Lyme disease. She approached me and asked about my symptoms. She shared that she also had Lyme disease that hadn't been diagnosed properly until eight years after she had contracted it. Judy also suffered from many cognitive problems. For the past five years, she had been under the care of Dr. Horowitz, a wonderful, progressive Lyme specialist. She told me that it might take several months to get an appointment with him, but she would do her best to help me. Two weeks later, a secretary from the doctor's office called Judy to schedule an appointment for me. It turned out that Judy had kindly written a letter about me and my illness to Dr. Horowitz and she had enclosed a copy of my book *Healing*. Dr. Horowitz was so generous to respond promptly.

When I went to see Dr. Horowitz for the first time, I was asked at the front desk to check off a list of possible symptoms. Speech difficulty was on the list, and so were difficulties with spelling, writing, concentration, and memory recall. My hearing was impaired at one point, as was my swallowing reflex so that I would choke on liquid and then on solid food. All the symptoms I recognized in myself were classic to those Lyme patients whose spirochetes had crossed the blood-brain barrier, gone into their brains and caused cognitive impairments and malfunctions of the cranial nerves, known as Neuro-Lyme. I had prepared my own History of Physical Illness (HPI), and I presented it to Dr. Horowitz, who then went through my personal medical history and wrote down my symptoms in his notes.

On the list of symptoms that I had filled out at the front desk, I had checked off urinary frequency. He asked me about it, and I told him that I was going to the restroom between twenty-five to thirty times during the day and five to seven times at night. He asked if I'd ever had it checked out. I said that I'd had some urinary frequency in medical school, but it became worse with low blood pressure and now with Lyme disease.

He went on to ask about my moods, whether I was experiencing depression or mood swings. I told him that it had caused me to be very weak physically, that there was so much pain everywhere in my body, and that I hardly had any energy in me.

I also described how I was experiencing my past all over again. As a nun, I had been able to transform a lot of my suffering, but with Lyme disease, these images arose again—not as strongly as I experienced them before—but they were vivid and powerful nonetheless. Certain images and emotions surged suddenly like a forest fire or a flood, and they could be overwhelming at times.

Dr. Horowitz listened attentively. He asked more questions about my neurological symptoms. He explained that when the Lyme bacteria, *Borrelia burgdorferi*, enter the brain, they release toxins that cause the outer layer of the nerves (the myelin sheath) to become inflamed and frayed, which results in headaches and cognitive dysfunction. The peripheral nerves are also damaged by the same mechanism, which causes pain, tingling, and numbness. In small as well as big joints, these toxins cause inflammation, which result in swelling and pain, notably migratory joint-pain. They also deposit in muscles and cause achiness and pain, like that in fibromyalgia.

He also said, "This Lyme disease is like a demon. Three-quarters of my Lyme patients relive their past experiences and past traumas. It's like a demon that digs into these experiences and makes them alive all over again."

When our mind is healthy or preoccupied, it can keep our mental experiences under control. It can also suppress certain thoughts, feelings, or past traumas, preventing them from manifesting at the conscious level.

However, when our body is sick, our mind also becomes more fragile and vulnerable. As a result, past suffering or unfinished business may surge uncontrollably to the surface.

I see that this phenomenon takes place not only in Lyme disease, but in other illnesses as well. When we have an acute illness, we experience fragility in our body. We may then start to worry whether we will be able to go back to work on time, or if we're sick too long, we may lose our job. If we have cancer or some kind of chronic illness, our past traumas may resurface and it can be very frightening.

Over the years, I have learned to sit quietly, be mentally present and not try to cover up whatever arises. This helps me to create a container for these strong emotions and thoughts, to look at them at a deeper level, and to heal them. During the most difficult period of my Lyme disease thus far, I didn't fear death, but as I observed the decline in my concentration and cognitive functions, my greatest fear was to lose my intelligence. After all, most of us identify ourselves with our intelligence, talents, and capacities. What would become of me then?

QIGONG PRACTICE

I learned qigong from Sister Binh Nghiem during the US Tour 2011, and I practiced it three times daily, each time for more than an hour, during that winter. I also exercised my arms every day for about forty-five minutes, swinging them rapidly backward and forward two thousand times each session, known as *dich can kinh*, to help increase blood circulation and reduce the pain I was experiencing in my left shoulder and left arm. I also practiced Touching the Earth. Sometimes I would exercise intermittently up to a total of five hours a day.

I could not practice sitting meditation for long, because my mind became drowsy, dispersed, or easily overwhelmed. Exercising was something I could do actively for myself, and I also used it to train my mind to anchor in my breathing and in my body. The breath and the body are real and dynamic; they serve as concrete objects of concentration for the mind to dwell upon.

In our little room, we had fresh orchids and candlelight. We burned sandalwood incense or sage often to enjoy its pleasant fragrance and to purify the air. We also had a small water fountain in the room and as I did qigong, I could hear the drops of water falling. All this helped me to be in touch with and aware of my five senses and to be in tune with the surrounding environment, instead of getting lost in my own thoughts and feelings such as sadness, fear, and anxiety.

It's necessary to do exercise regularly and at a regular time, so that it becomes an integral part of our body.

As I continued to gain my physical strength and endurance, I also began to do jumping rope and then swimming. In jumping rope, I would breathe in and do five jumps, breathe out and do five jumps, counting up to three thousand jumps during forty-five minutes. In swimming, I would follow my in-breath while my head was above the surface of the water and follow my out-breath while my head was under the water. The different exercises I have been doing help increase blood circulation, ameliorating the symptoms and allowing me to cope better with the pain and to sleep somewhat more easily. Because I stay with my breathing and keep track with the counting, I also train my concentration so that it becomes stronger, instead of deteriorating as a result of the neurological Lyme disease.

During the first winter at Blue Cliff, my sisters were also kind to massage me when I really needed it. The Vietnamese herbal doctor told me that massaging the painful areas and spooning (*cao gio*, scrubbing the skin gently with the spoon) along the spine were good for the blood flow, and the human contact itself was also essential. When we're unwell, we can become isolated and withdrawn, and so we lack human contact and human touch. When we open up to receive help from others, it's an opportunity to feel connected with family members and, in my case, with my monastic sisters.

In the world, even when we have our spouses and children around us, most of the time when we're sick, we resort to painkillers and other drugs. However, no miracle drugs can take the place of our loved ones. Even if we're in a coma or on the deathbed, our beloved can still massage our feet and our hands. This human love remains important to us until the very last breath.

TOUCHING THE EARTH

I was aware that if I didn't take care of my body and keep it physically fit, my mind would continue to weaken, and then my body would become weaker too. The mind and body affect one another.

My mindfulness and concentration, instead of faltering during the course of my illness, has actually become stronger than before thanks to the mindfulness practices, qigong, and other exercises. This in turn helped me to detect the early symptoms of cognitive dysfunction and to correct promptly the mistakes I was making in my thinking, my speech, and my writing.

I am thankful to have had the good habit of exercising regularly since high school. In college, I swam slowly but steadily for up to an hour and thirty minutes at a time. I also jogged and lifted weights throughout my college and medical school years. I continued to jog and go hiking frequently since becoming a nun. These habits have helped me to have the self-discipline, physical strength, and endurance to go through the difficult times in my life.

Many young people nowadays lead a sedentary life style, and they don't have the habit of taking good care of their bodies. When they're sick, they rely mainly on medications, or they may sleep all day just to forget the discomforting physical and psychological symptoms. This kind of sleep is neither restful nor healing; it can result in nightmares, further lethargy, and depression.

Although the weather was bitterly cold that winter, besides doing qigong, I would go to the meditation hall and do 108 prostrations. I did each one slowly.

The first time I did this Touching the Earth practice, just naturally, an image from the past came to my mind—and this happened each time I touched the Earth in that session. It was an image about something unskillful I had done to myself or another person. For the 108 times of

Touching the Earth, more than 108 memories arose of times that I had been unskillful, either recently or long ago in the past.

When each image arose, I would touch the Earth and say, "Please forgive me; I didn't know better." I would begin anew with myself and release the unskillful action into the Earth, touching forgiveness and healing in myself. Then I stood up stably and breathed, and as I came down to touch the Earth again, another memory would spontaneously appear and I would practice beginning anew with myself again.

The second time I went to the meditation hall for this practice of Touching the Earth, the unskillful actions that I had done with my body would arise—the way I had thrown things or moved my body or walked away violently, or the way I had neglected or abused my own body or put it in dangerous or risky situations. Those images would arise spontaneously, and again I would apologize to myself and to the people involved, and I would forgive myself every time I touched the Earth.

The practice came naturally to me that way, and it brought an incredible sense of lightness and healing.

The third time I went to do Touching the Earth, at one point, it came to me that the tick that bit me and gave me Lyme disease had Buddha nature within it. As I was lying on the Earth, the thought came to me that both the tick and I had Buddha nature; therefore the tick can live inside of my body and we can be in harmony with each other!

The common view and approach to illness is that we must eliminate the bacteria or remove the tumor from our body in order to regain our health.

The discovery—that we can live in harmony with the virus, the bacteria or the tumor; that we can accept, take care, and live with each other in harmony—is definitely a wonderful possibility. This approach can help remove the feeling of fear, aversion, rejection, or hatred toward our sickness and toward our own body.

That moment when I saw that the tick had Buddha nature and that I could live in harmony with it in my own body was a moment of deep healing. I had listened to my Teacher talking about the Buddha nature not only in human beings but also in animals, plants, and minerals, but it was something different when I myself touched that insight in a moment of quietude, calm, and spaciousness of my own body and mind. That insight arose to me directly, fresh and clear.

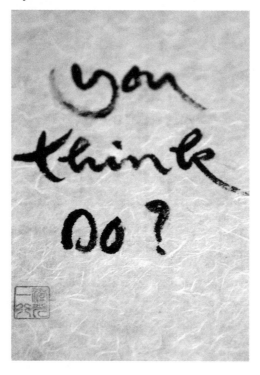

TICK IN THE DREAM

That same week I also had an amusing and enlightening dream. I was talking to a young woman with long blond hair, and I saw something on her hair that looked like a worm, fluorescent green, very fat, almost half the size of my little finger. I tried to flick it gently from her hair, but it wouldn't budge, so I tried again. On the third try, I flicked it forcefully and it flew out of her hair. In my dream, I tried to justify this harsh action by saying, "This tick can kill you!" I said it with a strong conviction and fear.

As I was saying it, I saw to my right side an entrance into a forest, and the tick was right there, so incredibly chubby and cute and green. It was about to walk into the forest, but before doing so, it turned sideways to look at me with a mischievous smile, and it winked at me!

I chuckled. I had just said "This tick can kill you!" but now a second thought came, "Well, it doesn't have to be such a big deal. I don't have to make a big deal out of this!"

This humor and friendliness was a moment of connection between me and the tick. I could laugh at myself and at my own fear toward the tick. I woke up from the dream with a smile. I told Sister Blue Sky about my dream and asked her, "You can draw Pooh Bear and the little Piglet very well. Would you draw this tick for me?" I explained how plump this tick was, and described the green color, and the smirk on its face.

My sister looked at me strangely, but she drew it for me anyway, and it was the cutest thing. I put the drawing up on the wall by my bed box and every time I took my medication, I would look at the tick and see it winking at me. I would say to it, "Help me to live in harmony with you. Help me to have no fear and to take care of you inside of me," and that became a practice for me.

TAKING MEDICATIONS

Dr. Horowitz is an internationally known specialist in Lyme disease. A consultation with him can cost almost one thousand dollars, and yet he has been seeing me for free this past two-and-a-half years. He also provided my medicine for free the first two years. Dr. Quang in Vermont, a Vietnamese herbal specialist, has also offered our brothers and sisters medicine for several years now. I have been taking medicines from both doctors, and they gradually help to strengthen the organs in my body and to remove the bacteria slowly from my bloodstream. So far, my illness isn't curable, but at least it can be kept under control with these medicines.

The triple antibiotics that I took for three months caused several side effects, and a part of me feared and resisted taking them. I also had to take probiotics to replace the millions of bacteria wiped out from my intestines daily. Sometimes the probiotic pills broke open in my throat, causing me to cough out a cloud of dry, smelly dust. Still, I would hold these pills in my hands, breathe, and recognize that these pills are bodhisattvas—they are great beings to help me heal.

I give rise to the awareness that there are many sick people who don't have access to medical care, and even those who do have access may not have the necessary stability in their home environment, bodies, or minds to take their medication. It isn't always easy to take medication daily on schedule. At certain points, I was taking medications ten times a day at specific hours, and I learned to appreciate the fact that one must have a clear and stable mind in order to go through this regimen.

From our first meeting, Dr. Horowitz recommended that I take more antibiotics. I had already taken two types of antibiotics and Plaquenil for three months and still suffered from ongoing side effects, including photosensitivity, jaundice, and tenderness in the liver area.

So I asked him, "Doctor, is it possible that I don't have to take antibiotics again? I don't think my body can take it anymore, and psychologically I can't take it anymore."

He was quiet for a moment and then said, "Sure, if you're not ready. We have developed very strong, concentrated herbal medicine that you can take."

Many people are turning to herbal medicine when they don't respond to antibiotics or they can't tolerate antibiotics long-term.

Dr. Horowitz went to another room, and when he came back, he told me that he had taken a moment to sit in silent contemplation and it came to him that the particular herbal medicines A-L complex and A-Bart complex might fit me well (for the Lyme bacteria as well as for the coinfection *Bartonella*, also known as cat scratch disease). He gave me a picture of the Buddha Medicine King and advised me, "When you take this medicine, remember to invoke the name of the Buddha of medicine. Then pray for the healing in other beings as well."

Since then, every time I take the medicine, I hold it quietly with both of my hands, breathe, and invoke three times: "Homage to the King

of Medicine, the King of Light, the One Who Comes from Suchness—
Nam Mo Duoc Su Luu Ly Quang Vuong Nhu Lai." I also evoke the
name of the Bodhisattva Avalokiteshvara, "The Great Being Who Listens
to the Cries of the World."

Then I pray, "Please help me heal the sickness and pain in my body.
Help me heal the wrong views, attachment, and despair in my mind. Thank
you for giving me the advantageous conditions to heal, and thank you for
giving me the capacity to heal. May I heal, and may I offer up this healing
without obstruction or hesitation to all other living beings. Whatever I
learn from this experience, I vow to share with others without obstruction
or hesitation."

Thus, I direct the energy of healing and love toward myself, and then
I direct it toward others. This gives me the inspiration and the aspiration
to heal not only myself but also others, and to offer the teachings I have
learned from my own experience.

The way we take our medications can influence our healing process.
Too often we take medications in a hurry while doing other things, or with
aversion or resistance toward the medication. At the moment we take the
medicine, if every thought of our mind is open to receive it and every cell
of our body is open to receive it, then even though we haven't swallowed
the pill, the whole process of healing has already begun.

On the contrary, if we resist our medication, we may have poor
intestinal absorption, and even when it's in the bloodstream it may not be
able to cross into the cells of our body. If the mind resists, the body will
not be able to receive it as effectively as it can.

According to the Buddhist teaching on the emptiness of transmission, the healer, the healed, and the healing process are not three separate entities, but they are in each other, and they are one. When I hold the cup of liquid herbal medicine in my two hands, I also visualize a forest of these herbal plants, of the people who tended them, harvested them and sent them to the United States, where they are transformed into concentrated drops of herbal medicine.

This experience is humbling because I see that the healing of my body and my mind involves innumerable beings, including the plants, the minerals, the doctors, my brothers and sisters, and lay friends, as well as the spiritual practice, time and space, and so on.

Sister Bamboo and Sister True Mind helped cook Dr. Quang's herbal medicines for me day after day these past two-and-a-half years. To see this amazing process that many humans, animals, plants, and minerals are involved in is to recognize that everything in the cosmos is involved in our healing.

MY SISTERS

Sister Bamboo and Sister Noble Truth lived with me in the same room during the first winter I stayed in Blue Cliff. They created conditions in the room to make it cozy, comfortable, accepting, and loving. The orchids in our room were healthy and beautiful, and often there were lit candles and burning incense. When I was so tired, the peaceful ambiance helped me feel comfortable lying down to rest or to sleep even if it was during the day. I didn't feel judged. I didn't feel expected to be active and vigorous.

I could exercise whenever I wanted, and I didn't feel awkward exercising in front of them.

My sisters brought food and drink to me when I could not go to the dining hall. When I moved to another room, sisters in my new room also cared for me. During the two years that I was seriously ill, my sisters and brothers in the monastery continued to take turns to cook, clean, and do office work and everything else. I didn't hold any particular responsibility. I had time and space to rest and to heal. I am grateful for these positive conditions.

I am aware that those of us living alone or with a small family may not have these conditions to stop, to rest, and to heal ourselves. When an animal is wounded, it doesn't chase after food or a mate anymore. It finds a safe place to lie down so that its body has a chance to rest and to heal.

As human beings, we have lost this capacity. We may be so numb or oblivious to our body that we aren't aware of the symptoms that are presenting themselves to us. Even when we know we're sick, we force ourselves to keep going. We take painkillers. We depend on adrenaline stimulated by our projects, pressure, and stress. We seek entertainment and diversion. We don't give our body a chance to rest and to heal itself until our illness becomes severe or we simply break down.

I am thankful to be a practitioner and to be able to stop and rest as a wounded animal would.

PRESENT MOMENT

Another important aspect of healing is the capacity to dwell in the present moment. During the worst part of my illness thus far, there were moments when despair arose strongly, but I breathed to calm down those waves of emotion. For the most part, mindfulness of my body and of my breathing has enabled me to dwell in the here and the now.

In the here and the now, I can recognize the good conditions available to me, such as a safe place to rest and heal in the presence and support of my sisters and brothers around me.

In the here and the now, I can continue to live my life fully and to experience beautiful memories with others. I learn to live in the moment as it is, and it helps me not to be burdened or plagued by my illness, by the past or by the future. Mindfulness allows you to be a child with wide open eyes, welcoming whatever arises.

Although the pain spread to more places and there were more neurological symptoms, mindfulness allowed me to be aware of the many conditions that were still positive and going well.

For example, the Neuro-Lyme disease impaired my cognitive functions, but it also stimulated a creative part of my brain. During the first winter at Blue Cliff, I wrote seven new songs that were joyful and meaningful. While I wasn't able to comprehend science and other complicated topics, I discovered I could memorize poetry easily. I memorized by heart quite a few epic poems written by Thay, which I hadn't been able to do before. In a way, I wish I had memorized Thay's entire book of poetry in Vietnamese; I probably could have done it, but I also practiced moderation since prolonged concentration caused me throbbing headaches. Also, I could comprehend and enjoy reading funny stories and legendary stories found in our library. Sister Boi Nghiem also brought me a book by Hans Christian Andersen from Magnolia Grove Monastery. I would chuckle or laugh out loud as I was reading it.

I would bring my guitar and the songs I wrote to the meditation hall and sing to myself. The joints in my fingers were swollen, so it was painful to play the guitar. I would have to put the guitar down often and take a few breaths, because both of my hands would be stiff, burning, and trembling uncontrollably. Still, I continued to play the guitar and, in fact, I played it more often than I ever did before, because I simply didn't want to lose this capacity.

I learned to take in only positive news. I said to my roommates, "I am sick. If you hear unkind things said about me or about anybody, or if there are stressful situations in the community, please help me by not bringing that kind of news into our room." Thus, my sisters helped nourish me with only joyful and positive stories, and I practiced nourishing my mind with positive thoughts and insights. I also continued to care for my sisters in my best capacity.

We often emphasize only the end result of an experience. In truth, the process of the experience is also extremely important. For example, if we go through an illness with a lot of sadness, anger, denial, or fear, then that experience is encoded in our memory as traumatic.

While the experience is happening, these negative emotions will affect the way the mind takes care of the body, the way the body will cope with the situation, and later, as we look back on the experience, we will most likely recall it as traumatic. This can cause the body to go through the whole trauma again both physiologically and psychologically.

If we continue to recall the experience as something negative or traumatic, then it's encoded in our long-term memory as such. When we experience something for the first time it's encoded in our short-term memory, but as we experience it mentally again and again, then it's encoded in our long-term memory, and that will later affect how we see our lives and how we cope with future situations.

Memory is found to be processed and stored in the hippocampus of the brain. In some studies on people with a normal hippocampus, subjects are asked to envision what the future will be like. It has been found that people use their past experiences to envision their future, meaning they project their past experiences onto the future. If the future is envisioned through the lens of the past and if the present moment is not well taken care of, then it becomes a negative past and when we think of the future, we will see it also as bleak and negative. Therefore, the way we take care of ourselves in every moment has a long-lasting effect.

JOY AND LAUGHTER

The antibiotics I was on for three months during the US Tour in 2011 made me more hyper than usual, but mindfulness helped that energy to manifest as joy and laughter. During the US Tour, I spent a lot of personal time with other sisters. We would drink tea and share childhood stories or joyful anecdotes. I wrote a joyful song called "Drink Your Tea!" and two of my younger sisters danced to it. Although four of us stayed in a small room—two slept on the bed boxes and two slept on the floor—we felt so comfortable and happy together.

Joy and laughter have been important to my healing. Sometimes when we're very sick or we experience a traumatic event, our mind can be so dark and bleak that we never want to think about it again. I feel that I have overcome the worst part of my illness, and I am now in the recovery process. When I look back to the three-month US Tour and the three winter months following that, I actually recall a lot of joy, laughter, creativity, sisterhood, and brotherhood. I continue to be nourished by that time.

Thus, it's important to create a healthy environment in which we offer and receive support when we're well and when we're sick. We also need to have a spiritual dimension in our lives in order to cultivate clarity and stability of mind, so we can continue to rejoice in life and see the conditions of happiness that we still have. Joy and lightness help nourish and heal our body and mind. If we're lost in loneliness, anxiety, and depression, we deprive ourselves of the opportunity to heal. Learning to dwell in the present moment, to be in the here and now, is an important practice when we're healthy. When we're sick, our mind and body are weakened, but if our mindfulness practice is already strong and supported by those around us, we're able to come back and dwell in the present moment more easily.

SISTER NOBLE TOOTH

It is our tradition to switch rooms before we start the Winter Retreat. Sister Noble Truth moved in to room with me and Sister Bamboo. On our first night together as roommates, when we were all quiet and about to fall asleep, Sister Noble Truth whispered in the dark, "May I read a poem to you?"

Sister Bamboo and I were so surprised and happy that even though it was already time for Noble Silence, we said, "Yes, of course, please read the poem!" Her voice was clear and childlike, and it was the sweetest poem.

Then the next night came, and as we were about to fall asleep, Sister Noble Truth whispered again, "Elder sister, will you read a poem for me?" I replied without hesitation, "Sure!" So we began a new tradition. For the rest of the winter, every night I would read a poem to her before she slept. If she was still tossing and turning, I would read another and then another, and often I would recite poetry for fifteen or twenty minutes into the night.

This inspired me to learn more poetry and to review the poems I already knew, because I didn't want to read her the same poems every night. This poetry reading helped my sister fall asleep more easily. Later, she confided in me that when the monastic brothers and sisters were violently evicted out of Bat Nha Monastery in Vietnam in 2009, many of them became traumatized by that experience. She had developed insomnia, and when she came to Blue Cliff Monastery, she continued to have this problem, but when I read poetry to her she could fall asleep easily. It was calming, soothing, and healing for her to hear my poetry and Thay's poetry.

This also gave me the opportunity to exercise my memory and to soothe myself before I went to sleep. So it became a meditation for the three of us every night to listen to poetry; occasionally, Sister Bamboo would read a poem also. This became a supportive condition for all three of us to heal.

Sister Noble Truth was twenty-one years old that winter—innocent, joyful, and also wise. Once she introduced her name to a lay practitioner, but the woman mistook her pronunciation for "Sister Noble Tooth." Since then, I would occasionally call her "Sister Noble Tooth." She followed all of the Sangha activities and played with sisters of her age during the day, and then when she came home at night, she would ring the wind chime outside and chant, "I have come under the lotus throne of the Buddha," to announce her arrival.

The truth was we could already hear her approach from two doors away, singing and laughing joyfully. Sister Bamboo and I usually tried to finish our bedtime routines early because we knew as soon as Sister Noble Truth entered the door, we would be laughing together.

Sometimes Sister Bamboo was gargling salt water or sesame oil and she would run into the bathroom to spit it out when Sister Noble Truth happened to come home early. Sister Bamboo would even try to gargle sesame oil an hour early and still Sister Noble Truth would appear suddenly and catch her. Sister Bamboo would have to discontinue her routine and she exclaimed, "I try to do it early, and you still come home unexpectedly!"

We would put everything aside, ready to hear about her day, which she recounted with great liveliness, humor, and insight. We tried to whisper and suppress our laughter because this was usually during Noble Silence. At times, the sisters next door or upstairs complained about our laughter, our giggles, or my reading of poetry late at night. I would apologize to them, but then it inevitably happened again.

I had been known as a solemn and serious person. I had always adhered to the practice of Noble Silence, and many times I didn't hesitate to remind others if they violated it. In the past, some sisters were afraid of me because I would practice it so strictly. However, as I became sick, I found myself relaxing and loosening up a lot more, actively generating joy inside myself, welcoming and accepting the joy that came from my sisters. It helped me to maintain myself as a flowering plant, open to receive water for growth and healing.

When we have physical and mental pain, it's easy to dry up due to our own irritation, agony, and despair, and if we become stuck in that state, our health, as well as our relationships with others, deteriorates quickly.

THRIVING ORCHIDS

There were some orchid plants in our room. Other rooms had them too, but it was amazing how those in our room constantly gave new blossoms as the old ones died. We believed that the orchids were thriving on our joy and laughter, and that our energy from doing qigong also fed the orchids.

It has been known that the green color of plants can instill calmness and peace in us, and I am sure that beautiful flowers can inspire joy, awe, and energy in us as well.

Conversely, our own energy can penetrate and affect plants. In nursing homes, elderly people are encouraged to take care of plants, because they become happier and healthier than those people who don't. The plants, also, are stronger when they're talked to and cared for as friends, instead of just receiving water routinely.

Nature provides us the great energy of peace and healing. Most monasteries, including ours, are founded in nature for this reason. As soon as people arrive, they feel relaxed and at ease, even though they may not know anything about the practice yet.

In our modern time, most of us live and work in big cities. Those in the helping professions and legal professions can be engrossed in the suffering of other people, all day long and year after year, and this takes place within concrete walls that appear impersonal, rigid, and lifeless. We need to be in touch with nature more frequently, so we may breathe in the fresh air, release our tensions and stale thoughts, touch joy, and heal ourselves from the traumas we've absorbed from others.

PLAYING ON A FROZEN LAKE

It snowed for a few days and the lake became frozen. One day during walking meditation I was at the tail end of the Sangha, and I stopped Sister Noble Truth and told her to stay behind with me. She looked at me with wide eyes when I told her, "We can skate on the ice! I'll pull you, okay?"

Neither she nor I had ever played this game before. First, I stepped on the ice slowly to see if it was thick enough. It looked and felt very thick, so I told her to lie down and I began to drag her out onto the frozen lake.

Sister Noble Truth screamed, "Elder sister, the tick in you is so strong!" I pulled her to the middle of the lake, and we lay down and looked at the clear blue sky, breathing and being quiet next to each other.

Then she tried to drag me back, but she was tumbling and falling. When we got back to shore, we decided that it was too much fun to leave the place, so I dragged her back out again. We lay down and enjoyed the blue sky for a long time.

In the midst of my illness, there were many joyful and meaningful moments like this one, and so when I look back to that time, it's not traumatic. Living fully in the present moment has given me wonderful memories and insights that continue to nourish me for years to come.

IMPERMANENCE

Being in touch with nature enlightens us to the fact that everything is in constant flux, such as the aging process that's constantly taking place within us. Even in the most beautiful leaf or flower, there is already at least a brown spot or a hole.

Seeing this impermanence, sickness, and aging in nature can help us recognize the same process in ourselves, reflect upon it, and accept it gradually. If we fail to do this—confining ourselves within concrete walls and being engrossed in our intellectual work day after day—we may see ourselves as fixed and unchanging in body and mind.

In this way, we may not appreciate the fact that, while each moment is passing, we are at that moment at the youngest age of the remainder of our lives, even if we're now twenty, thirty, fifty or even eighty. To be in touch with our youth and our health is to be aware of impermanence, rejoicing and taking good care of the positive conditions available to us.

Even if there are dysfunctions in our body, we can still be in touch with what is going right within us. If we've been stuck in a rigid and stifling place, physically and mentally, then we will be surprised on the day when we suddenly look at ourselves, asking, "Since when did I grow old? How have I aged? What has happened to my body? What has happened to my mind? How have I become such an angry person, a sad person, or a bitter person? Who am I?"

Aging and changes in personality take place day by day, moment to moment. It's just like when a tumor is diagnosed; that tumor has already been there for a few years before an MRI or a CT scan could detect it.

As a result of my illness, my body has been aging much more quickly. I had seen one brown spot on my right hand for three years, but just during that last winter alone, when I was most sick, I saw one spot after another appearing. They weren't as dark as the first one, but if I turned my hand at a certain angle, I could see many more of them. In fact, all the brown spots were already there, and it was just a matter of time and health conditions until they manifested more or less obviously.

RATTLESNAKE

Nature has a healing quality, and it also helps us to come back and reflect upon ourselves and to accept who we are and where we are.

I observed signs of aging on my face as well. One day I saw two spots that seemed to have appeared on my face overnight. It became an obsession to look at these age spots and to wish they were gone.

Then a memory came to me. On one Lazy Day at Deer Park Monastery, a group of brothers and sisters decided to go hiking together and to look for the waterfall that we had discovered the winter before. We decided to find the waterfall from the top down this time. We were crawling under bushes one after another, because there was no trail for a while. Sometimes we would turn around and look at each other and smile brightly.

Here we were—all Dharma teachers—and we were like children joyfully crawling under the bushes. We ended up somewhere that was so thick in the forest that we couldn't see anything. One brother was assigned to climb up a tree and look out to see where we were and to find the direction of the waterfall. He actually saw it from afar, and we continued in that direction.

We crossed through poison oak thickets, and by this point, there was no return. I talked to the poison oak, "Please forgive me. I mean no harm, so please don't harm me." Amazingly enough, none of us suffered from it. We eventually made it to the top of the waterfall, and we were so exhausted that each one of us found a spot and fell fast asleep.

When I woke up, I started to walk among the rocks and stopped dead when I saw a gigantic rattlesnake, with beautiful brownish coloring, hanging from a cave and leaning toward the branch of a tree. One brother was lying directly beneath the snake, which was only a few feet above him.

The rattlesnake sensed my presence, made a rattling sound, and moved back into the cave. Simultaneously, my brother heard the rattling, got up, and jumped off to the side.

Later, as I was looking at myself in the mirror and trying to reconcile with the two new spots I had just discovered on my face, I thought that the intense moment with the snake hanging above my brother could have caused these spots!

These spots are marks of time, and they are the marks of my life. In my life, I have gone through joyful and loving as well as painful experiences, and they all leave their marks on my face and on my body.

If I wanted my body to remain youthful, impeccable, and perfect, then would I be willing to remove these marks of time and the experiences of my life? I am because of these experiences. I don't want to deny them or to deny this process in my own body. Looking at aging in this light, I have learned to be more affectionate toward the changes in my own body, and to be accepting, loving, and at peace with them.

To recognize the freckles and brown spots on my face and hands is to learn to breathe through waves of despair and fear, to observe this phenomenon in nature more closely, and to acknowledge that aging is happening even in a child or a young person. Sitting at the breakfast table, I hold up an apple to appreciate how beautiful and delicious it looks, and as I continue to look at it, I see brown spots on it. However fresh and perfect it may appear, it's already in the process of aging. The same is true of a banana. Even when it's still greenish-yellow, there are many black and brown spots on it already. Learning to recognize and to smile to the impermanence and aging in the apple, the banana, and all natural phenomena is to familiarize ourselves with, and make peace with, this process in our own bodies.

FOREWARNING SIGNS

I have also learned about the course of my illness and aging process from my sleep. Many nights I'm awakened by a sharp pain in my body. I may not feel the pain in that particular place during the day, but it manifests at night.

For example, when I was taking the triple antibiotics, I would wake up with pain under my ribs, in the right upper quadrant of my abdomen. Sometimes the pain was so severe that my body doubled over. I would put my right hand on that area and breathe with the waves of pain in order to be with it and to relax it. I prayed to the Buddha or to Mother Earth, or I simply told myself, "It's okay, it's okay, my love," until I could fall back to sleep again.

There was also a raging fire in some of my dreams. I told my sister about these incidents, and she said probably my liver was "hot." Slowly, my skin and eyes began to look jaundiced. Later when I went to see Dr. Horowitz and had blood tests done, many of them came back abnormal, including all eight enzymes in my liver function test.

At night, I also experienced pain in certain joints in my arms and legs that were apart from the places that I experienced during the day. I returned to my mindful breathing in order to calm my body as well as my mind. Anxiety, fear, and sorrow only worsen the pain and further complicate the course of the illness. From the nightly dreams and pain, I discovered that the seed of our illness is already present in our body, and if our sleep is light enough and our mind is calm and alert enough, we can recognize the latent symptoms during the night. These symptoms will eventually surface in our daily lives, but if we can detect them early during the night, then we can take better care of ourselves. As long as our mind remains clear and stable, we have the confidence that we will be able to take care of our body and to accept what is to come.

ACKNOWLEDGING IMPROVEMENTS

Another important part of healing is to be able to be aware of the improvement and the progress we make. When we see that one symptom improves, however minor it may be, we should be able to recognize it and acknowledge it.

Mindfulness enables us to be more sensitive and aware of the changes in our own body. For example, I have developed neuropathic pain along my two arms because when the bacteria go into the bloodstream, they secrete toxins that are toxic to the myelin sheaths of the neurons, causing them to become inflamed, frayed, and torn, so there is pain as well as interruption of the nerve conduction. The same process takes place in the brain in Neuro-Lyme disease, resulting in cognitive dysfunction. It's often difficult for me to fall asleep and to sleep without frequent interruption because of the headache and the pain in my arms and joints. I exercise daily to help increase blood circlation, and maintain joint flexibility and muscular strength. I mentally scan through my body frequently, acknowledging the painful and pain-free elements:

As I follow my in-breath and out-breath, I scan through each part of my body, and I smile to each part of my body.

As I follow my in-breath and out-breath, I am aware of pain in a particular part of my body. I smile and relax that part of my body. I am here. I am here for this pain, my dear.

As I follow my in-breath and out-breath, I am aware that there is no pain or less pain in a particular part of my body. I smile with gratitude to that part of my body. Thank you, thank you, my dear.

As I follow my in-breath and out-breath, I am aware that my body and mind are still whole and intact. I give rise to happiness and gratitude that my body and mind are still whole and intact.

I scan through my body in this manner frequently throughout the day, relax tension, and give thanks to the parts not affected or that are doing better at the moment. I also apply this scanning method to my thoughts, feelings, perceptions, and attitudes. Because this disease has affected my cognitive functions, I often ask myself, "Am I thinking logically? Are my thoughts in line with right views? Am I reluctant to do something because I don't really like it, or is it because of the new limitations from my illness?" These questions help me acknowledge thoughts, feelings, perceptions, or attitudes with more spaciousness and distance, so as not to blindly identify myself with them.

Another symptom that I practiced with was the shortness of breath caused by Lyme disease. During walking meditation, I could only take one step with each breath. If I tried to prolong my breath and took more steps, I felt suffocated, and my body tensed up. My lung capacity could only allow one step per in-breath, and one step per out-breath. Sometimes even that was tiring.

On Lazy Days, I went walking slowly on a two-mile loop with severe shortness of breath. That loop wouldn't have been anything when I was in Deer Park Monastery, where I climbed up on mountains and rocks the entire Lazy Day. Now at Blue Cliff Monastery, just walking on level land seemed effortful and exhausting.

Still, Sister Bamboo and I went walking on most Lazy Days. I also exercised daily to maintain physical fitness. All of these consistent efforts helped not only my body but also my mental well-being. Slowly I recognized that there was an improvement. On walking meditation, I could take four steps when I breathed in and four steps when I breathed out, and for the most part it didn't feel tiring or exhausting.

My mind could dwell with my breath and my steps. As spiritual practitioners, we're fortunate to have such tools to measure our improvements concretely, and when we have a small improvement, we need to recognize and acknowledge it, which in turn reinforces our faith in our capacity to transform and to heal in body and mind.

Awareness of the interbeing nature between the body and the mind enables us to accept what comes with more equanimity. Ordinarily, when we feel or think something, we immediately conclude that this is how and what we are, and we identify ourselves with these thoughts and feelings.

Closer observation reveals that body and mind affect one another, and they manifest in each other. So in the course of illness, we have to be very careful not to identify ourselves with our symptoms. This practice frees us from overwhelming fear and despair, saving up energy that we can use to heal ourselves.

For example, I noticed that I kept gaining weight even though I didn't eat more than usual. I also experienced melancholy and bouts of depression frequently. Later the blood tests revealed that I had low levels of thyroid hormones. It turned out that Lyme disease impaired the function of my thyroid gland, and Dr. Horowitz confirmed that most Lyme patients suffered from hypothyroidism. It slowed down my metabolism and triggered depression and lethargy. I had to take thyroid hormone replacement, which caused anxiety, tachycardia, and palpitation even at a very low dose. It was so uncomfortable, and I had to relax my body and reassure myself, "It's okay, there's nothing to be anxious about. It's only the effects of the medication." Thankfully, after about six months, my thyroid level returned to a low normal range, and I was able to discontinue the medication.

My cognitive functions such as speech, memory recall, reading skills, and writing skills were also impaired. I had to breathe to calm down the waves of fear of losing my intelligence. Because the practice helped me to stay calm and aware, I was able to detect the errors I was making in pronunciation, word choice, spelling, etc. Then I promptly corrected these errors. I did this again and again for myself even when my sisters didn't seem to notice or mind the mistakes I was making. Thanks to my own patience toward myself, I have been able to recover most of these cognitive functions. It's only when I'm extremely tired or burdened by another sickness, like a cold, that these symptoms become more salient again. Dr. Horowitz had informed me that cognitive functions would take a long time to recover, and only partially at times. About one year into my illness, when he saw my expeditious progress, Dr. Horowitz exclaimed "It's a miracle!" three times.

It is essential during illness to be aware of the improvements as well as the active symptoms, because sometimes we're so drowned in our pain, fear, or depression that even when there's some improvement we don't recognize it or refuse to acknowledge it because it seems minimal or fleeting.

When we first become sick, our loved ones offer us much attention and care. However, in chronic illness, the amount of attention and care we receive may become less and less, because our friends and loved ones have to move on to take care of things for themselves and for us.

We may identify ourselves with our own illness, feeling lonely and isolated, and if we aren't careful, we may feel neglected or deserted. Our expectation that people should have empathy for us and pay attention to us can lead to severe disappointment, and we can become bitter and needy, grasping on to people and pushing them away at the same time.

In practicing mindfulness of our body and mind, we give ourselves the attention and love we need and we take care of ourselves moment to moment, so that we don't need so much from others. We also learn not to identify ourselves with our illness; this illness is a part of us, but it is not everything about us. There is ill-being in certain parts of our body, but there is well-being in the rest of our body as well.

We should be able to rejoice in the wellness of our being, physically and mentally. We definitely don't have to play the role of a sick person for attention or pity.

In the end, I have realized that even though there are those who love me dearly, no one can suffer my physical or mental pain and no one can heal my body and my mind. Even though my Teacher, my monastic brothers and sisters, my own blood brother, and my friends have faith in my practice and give me many positive conditions, I still must be the one responsible for my own healing, taking advantage of the opportunities at hand in order to heal myself.

It is important to continue to live fully and to rejoice in the conditions of happiness and improvement available to us, which give us further strength and energy to take better care of ourselves. When we acknowledge the body, the body responds to us. When we have faith in the healing capacity of our body, our body heals better. Although there may be damaged organs in our body, although there may be pain in many parts of our body, although there may be sadness and despair in our feelings, we may still be able to say to ourselves, "My body and mind are still whole and intact. Thank you for still being intact."

It is a great happiness to be able to say this to ourselves, because we know that our love is still intact. We continue to be there for ourselves no matter what.

THE CICADA

There is a Zen story about a cicada. One day a young man walks by a forest and hears a cicada crying. The sound is heartbreaking. The young man asks the cicada, "What happened? Why are you crying like this?" The cicada replies, "My wife just died and I don't know how I will live the rest of my life."

The young man considered that a cicada's life is only twenty-four hours long, and it was already midday; there were less than twelve hours left of the cicada's life, but nevertheless it felt that there was so much time left that it didn't know how it would be able to manage it.

The life span of a human might be one hundred years, but it's like twenty-four hours compared to the Earth or the sequoia that can live three thousand years. Our life span is only like the life of a cicada, and yet we want to end our lives when we experience despair in illness or trauma.

To see that our life is so short and fragile, and yet so amazing, we learn to be more careful with our thoughts and speech and bodily actions. We learn to accept what is and to cherish this life, which is brief and precious.

Lately, when I lie down in bed, I visualize myself as a cicada. When I imagine myself in the body of Sister Dang Nghiem, it feels large, taking up the whole bed box, but there's something humbling and comforting to me to see myself in the size and shape of a cicada, this little brown thing lying on the immense Earth.

I say to Mother Earth, "Mother, I come back to you, and I take refuge in you. Please hold the pain and tension in my body and mind, and help me heal. If I were to die tonight, I know I am just going back to you. You have brought me to life, and you have given me this body. I am going back to you every moment, and when this body disintegrates, I go back to you entirely so that I may come forth again." It gives me peace to breathe and evoke the capacity to heal in me and in Mother Earth. I entrust myself to Mother Earth to embrace and heal me, and if I were to go this night, I would be at peace.

IMPACT OF SUICIDAL MESSAGES

When I experienced depression or despair in the past, I simply wished to kill myself. Since the time I was nine years old, I had been haunted by death. I would stand on the rail of any bridge, looking down at the water and visualizing myself plunging in and losing myself in the water. I took a handful of pills with the intention to end my life when I was fifteen years old. As an adult I also entertained that thought frequently, and when I became a nun, that thought continued to arise.

However, with mindfulness, I have learned to speak to my death wish every time it arises, "One day I will die. In fact, this body is dying and being reborn each moment. I don't have to wish for death. Just live beautifully and die beautifully each moment." Sometimes I also say to myself, "As long as I still wish to die, I am still caught in the notion of birth and death."

Over the years of practice, this death wish comes to me less frequently, even when I have difficulties in myself. Whenever it did arise, I would just smile to it and breathe with it, and it would vanish. However, during the first winter at Blue Cliff Monastery, with my cognitive functions being so impaired and the physical pain relentless and unbearable at times, I experienced despair in strong waves.

Then, for the first time in my life, I realized I had been so unskillful all these years in wishing myself to die. I had given every cell of my body this message to die; and it had become my habit to resort to thoughts of death every time I faced a serious problem in my life. When we send a powerful message like that to our body—that we don't want to live any more, that we want to destroy our body—it shakes the whole body and each cell to the core. The life energy in us becomes dimmer, and we are walking around more like a corpse.

Even though I was only forty-three years old, my body wasn't able to fight off the Lyme disease perhaps because for too many years I wished my body to be destroyed and to disappear, and this message has had a severe impact on it. My body was able to withstand this impact over the years, but it has become weakened, and now it's no longer able to function and to protect me as effectively.

I hope that young people become more aware of the messages that you are sending to your body. Learn to cherish this life and evoke life in every cell of your body. Express confidence in your body and in its capacity to heal and transform.

Journal Entry

April 19, 2013

A few days ago during morning sitting meditation, I sat with my yearning again. It is an expansive feeling that has a twinge of bitter sweetness. As usual, I quietly breathe with its waves. Then in my mind, an image of a queen in her palace appears. Amidst the grandeur and beauty of the physical world around her, she is alone with her own loneliness and her death.

Then an image of a person with many children surrounding him arises in my mind. He, too, is writhing alone in his final moments.

Many images of that nature continue to manifest in my mind. I recognize that I, too, will always have to face my own loneliness and my own death. No one can bear its weight for me, no matter how much the person may love me. Then the image of me lying on my deathbed arises. My yellow Sanghati robe gently drapes over my body from the neck down. There is a smile on my lips. Is there anyone next to me? It doesn't seem to matter to me. There is a smile on my lips, and that's all that matters.

In that moment, I touch lightness, peace, and acceptance within myself, for myself and my own life. May I continue to learn to love in the spirit of non-grasping. May I respect and protect my freedom and the freedom of those I vow to love. May we continue to be able to look each other in the eye. May we laugh together and count on each other. May there be a smile on our lips whenever we think of one another. May there be a smile on your lips in your last moments. May there be a smile on my lips in my last moments. May there be no more yearning or waiting.

LONELINESS AND YEARNING

During the course of my Lyme disease, I also experienced a deep loneliness and yearning. In Vietnamese there are two words *ai* and *duc*. "Ai" means attachment and "duc" means desire. They are often coupled together as ai duc to describe the sexual energy in us.

When we're sick, feelings of attachment can arise readily because we touch the fragility and impermanence of our body more keenly than ever before. Since most of us identify ourselves with our body, the fear of losing ourselves, via the loss of our body, becomes very strong. This fear is in everyone, but it's most haunting when we're severely sick or dying.

Even though I'm a nun, the need to have someone special in my life is still there. While I was so sick, this need became much stronger. I wished to have someone there to go through the experience with me, to care for me, to give me assurance, and last but not least, to remember me when I'm gone.

Waves of yearning and despair arose simultaneously. Beautiful past memories flooded my consciousness day and night. Although mindfulness helped remind me that I was blessed to be surrounded by kind and loving sisters, at times their presence didn't seem to be enough. I learned to smile to that thought.

As much as my own blood brother loved me, he could not afford to be near me and to take care of me. Again and again, I reminded myself to be grateful for all that I had, instead of feeling restless and searching for what I didn't have.

As I was in touch with my body and its fragility, I saw clearly that I don't have complete control over it. I take care of it the best way I can, but I also have to accept what would become of it.

If I cannot grasp my own body and make it the way I want it to be, then how can I grasp someone else's body? It is just not possible.

My mind is so much more elusive and abstract than my body. Feelings, thoughts, and perceptions come and go. If I cannot hold onto or grasp my own mind, then how can I hold onto or grasp another person's mind? Even if a person's mind is beautiful, I cannot hold onto it. Neither can I grasp that person's feelings, thoughts, and perceptions.

Thus, I have learned to confront my attachment and desire by constantly contemplating on my own body and mind. This helps me to be realistic and to come back to the fact that the only thing I can do is to take care of myself; I can't expect anyone else to do it for me, or to endure the physical and mental pain that I'm going through.

This realization also helps to alleviate the disappointment, frustration, and sadness that we tend to feel when we're fragile or vulnerable—at those times when we might expect others to understand and feel what we feel but they cannot. Our loved ones can only create positive conditions for us, but we ourselves must make use of those positive conditions to take care of ourselves.

Sexual desire too can arise strongly when we're physically and mentally weak and vulnerable. We desire to be loved and not to be forgotten. The way we absorb sexual messages via our six senses throughout our lives also affects our sexual energy and its manifestation during the course of our illness.

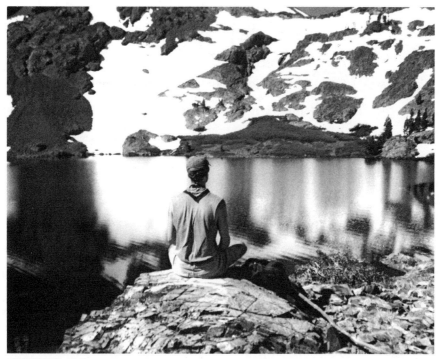

JOHN SEAVER, 1999

Nothing we consume and absorb is ever lost. It's deposited in our store consciousness, where it's processed and maintained. I have been in the monastery for almost fifteen years now, but sometimes during sitting meditation images that I have seen in movies years before will arise vividly. It seems as if the barrier between the store consciousness and the mind consciousness becomes more porous when we're sick, so that images of the past can arise more forcefully than ever. Breathe with those images and calm them down with mindful breathing. "Breathing in, I am aware that there is desire in me. Breathing out, I calm the desire with my out-breath." Bring stability and peace to our body posture. If instead we follow our sexual instincts, we can become needy and dependent on other people, and we may get involved in sexual relations that bring more sadness and destruction to our body.

Back when I was in medical school, some of the incarcerated youth I worked with at the youth guidance center in San Francisco said that if they contracted HIV, they would go out and have sex with as many people as they could. One reason for this was that they felt angry with the world, and they wanted to get revenge by spreading the illness. Another reason was that they felt frightened and utterly alone.

All of us wish to have a special connection with someone. When we're lonely or sick, we yearn even more desperately for this connection. However, when there's too much instability and suffering in us, we can never make a true connection. We can only bring more suffering to our body and mind, and this impedes our process of healing. Coming back to ourselves and taking care of our own body and mind is the deepest connection that we can make, and this serves as a strong foundation for us to relate to other people.

Many people work and get involved in relationships and projects in order to forget their illness or other crisis. Perhaps their problem will be covered up for a while, but it will come back and become even more severe.

As practitioners, we learn from every experience that we go through. If we allow ourselves to stop and look deeply into our illness, we will benefit so much from it.

We humans need to come back to this innate capacity, and simplify and prioritize our life. What is truly important? What do we really need to do? Then let go of those things that aren't so important. We may allow ourselves to take time off, to be home, to rest, to exercise, to eat a special diet, or to look for the appropriate doctors. It requires a lot of self-awareness, which will bring self-understanding and self-love and acceptance.

HEALING IN AGING AND DEATH

Loss of a Loved One

During childhood, I experienced many losses. I didn't know my father, but I was told that he was an American serviceman, and that he died in the Vietnam War. I last saw my mother when I was twelve years old. It was an ordinary day. My mother went to the market to tend to her clothing shop, and I still remember standing on the stairway looking at her as she was giving my grandmother money to buy food for the day. She wore a simple outfit, embroidered around the neck, the hem, and the wrists. Then my mother walked out of the house, and that was the last time I saw her.

Then, in 1985, I went to the United States, and a year later, my grandmother passed away, and then my uncle in 2003.

So I have had many deaths of my relatives during my life, but I think it was John's death in 1999 that affected me the most because he was my own partner. I was not there when John died. In fact, I was not physically present for any of these deaths—my father, my mother, my grandmother, my uncle, or John.

I had to face my own death directly after John died in an accident. He went to the ocean to swim, but before that, he was doing yoga on the beach. Some people saw him doing yoga. Something about him impressed them, so they watched him for a while. Then they continued on a long walk, and when they came back, they saw his clothes on the shore but didn't see him anywhere.

They looked for him. When it became late, but they still didn't see anyone out there in the water, they called the Coast Guard. Helicopters came to look for John. Policemen found his car, searched his clothes and saw his card, so they came to our house to look for us.

I was on duty at Oakland Children's Hospital. My best friend who lived right next door to us had received the news, so she came to Children's Hospital and paged me at two o'clock in the morning. I thought John had called to wish me a happy birthday, but as soon as I heard my friend's voice asking "Is that you, Huong?" I knew something very wrong had happened. I went out to the lounge to meet her, and my first question was, "What happened to John?"

I remember clearly everything that had already happened on the day John passed away. That morning I was driving from my apartment to the hospital in Oakland. It was about an hour's drive. At that time I had my own apartment in Martinez, where I was doing my residency. I would drive to Children's Hospital Oakland as a part of my rotation.

I had been driving through beautiful mountain scenery that sunny autumn morning. Everything was lush and bright. I had started thinking of John. Just three weeks before that, I had gone to the retreat of Thay;

and during the retreat, I realized how I had let the stress of work pull me away from our relationship.

When I came back from the retreat, I appreciated John much more deeply, and yet something in me withdrew from him. I didn't know how to come back to "normal" life after the retreat. While there, I had learned that if I practiced I could transform my suffering, but when I came back to my medical residency the stress was the same as before, and I also saw everything in a different light. Ignorance, in a way, had been bliss. This new awareness of my suffering and happiness made it even more isolating and more poignant for me to bear.

Right after the retreat I had been very inspired, but then I became depressed because I was not able to maintain the practice.

During my drive to the hospital that morning, I felt my deep joy and love for John all over again. He was my soul mate, and I wanted to do my best to take care of our relationship and not to lose him.

As I was driving into Oakland, I suddenly saw gigantic dark clouds enshrouding the area. It was a great contrast to be driving from a sunny bright day into a dark, foreboding city. I could hardly see the cars in front of me.

I thought to myself, "Life is also like this at times. The clouds can come in like this, but I have to remember that the sun is always there. It's actually just right behind me."

Throughout the day at the hospital I thought of John. I left him several messages letting him know that I thought of him, that I loved him and appreciated him, and wished him a good day. That was on September 25, 1999. The next day would be my birthday.

John had asked if we could spend my birthday together. I had told him I would be working, but in part I was avoiding him.

However, on that day, I sincerely wanted to connect with him again and to see him. At 2 a.m. the following morning, early on my birthday, when my friend Jennifer called me at work and asked, "Is that you, Huong?" I intuitively knew something had happened to John.

I went out to the lounge to talk to her, and we drove to the ocean. His two best friends and their girlfriends were already there. In the dark of the night, I was crying and howling as loudly as the ocean was. I begged, "Please take care of my loved one!" I was utterly small and in total despair. My whole world was turned upside down.

As we drove back home from the ocean, I said to my friend, "I'm not going back to medicine." She quietly replied, "I would understand."

I came home. I opened the door and turned on the light. The ambiance in the apartment was so light, gentle, and bright. He had spent the whole day cleaning the apartment, and he had washed all of our clothes and folded them neatly. Everything was in perfect order. Everything was calm and peaceful. I burst out crying. His presence was palpable. His love, his care, his peace, and his joy were all there. I had established an altar in our front room, with a photo of the Bodhisattva Avalokiteshvara standing while holding the bottle of the nectar of compassion. There were also photos of my mother and my grandmother, and an incense holder. I lit the incense and knelt down in front of the altar, holding the long stick until it burned completely.

My friend Jennifer was exhausted, so she slept near me on the sofa.

While I was kneeling like that, my mind was completely quiet. I wasn't suffering, and I wasn't thinking at all, even though I had never done meditation on my own.

John was the one who had done sitting meditation every night before we went to sleep. I just sat next to him, waiting for him to finish. I myself had never learned about meditation until I went to Thay's retreat three weeks earlier.

While I was kneeling, my mind was in a state of quietude and oneness. I felt that he hadn't left this room yet, and I could be there with him for the last time. After the incense burned completely, I turned around to look out the window. The sun had risen and sunlight was reflecting on the windows and the rooftops of houses at a distance from our apartment.

Our apartment was on Potrero Hill in San Francisco, so we could see the houses way below. The sun was reflecting on the windows in such a way that it formed a gigantic heart—not the heart you usually see on Valentine's cards, but an anatomical heart. I cried out loud, "John, I see you!" and the cry woke up my friend Jennifer.

John's death plunged me into deep despair. I had lost him. He was my soul mate who understood me and listened to me, who was there to be my friend to play and explore nature with me, to care for me as my partner, but he was also like a father and a mother to me.

He respected my choices and decisions, so whatever I wanted to do, he supported me wholeheartedly. For example, when I wanted to go to Kenya for three months, he asked me if I wanted him to go with me and I replied that I wanted to go alone. So he let me do so.

When I planned to go to Vietnam, again I said that I wanted to go alone, and he respected that. I had a lot of independence in our relationship, and we were close friends to each other. I lost that partnership in him. I lost that person who loved and cared for me—the love and care I hadn't received from my own father and mother.

Another reason John's death plunged me into deep despair was guilt. I had turned away from him and toward my sadness of the past. I would curl up with my depression and push him away during those periods.

This feeling of guilt haunted me and hurt me so. Most noticeably, his death made me face my own life and death. If I had loved somebody who didn't know how to love and care for himself and me, I probably would have just gone back to medicine and tried to make it through.

However, I had loved someone who lived beautifully and who died beautifully. The ocean was the place he loved most, and he had said to me a few times that if he ever died to please let his body be in the ocean; he wanted to die like the Alaskans, to be put in a little boat and pushed out to sea. In fact, the second night after John had died, in my dream I saw that I was floating in the ocean. My arms stretched out as far as they could, and so did my body. The water was completely still, crystal clear, and blue. A feeling of profound peace and calmness spread through my body and the water. That sensation lasted for a long time. When I woke up, I felt assured that John himself experienced this profound peace in the moment he let go.

John lived a short life, but a beautiful life, and he died the way he wanted to die. Even though it happened unexpectedly, he died the most beautiful death. He was not sick, and he was not torn by any sort of suffering at all. I know he was saddened by the state of our relationship, about how I was withdrawing, but he was handling it well.

John's death made me question everything I was doing. If I were to die in the midst of the day like John, could I say that I had lived a full and peaceful life? The answer was a definitive no. Could I go back to medicine? Could I go back to living in forgetfulness and in depression? I knew that the depression would be more severe than ever before. I had done it all my life, but it was because I had great ambitions and delusions. Now everything was shattered and raw, and the momentum was gone. I could not do it anymore.

I thought about committing suicide, but I knew I would never see him again because he would go in a different direction. Moreover, if I were to die, all the good things that I had done for my brother and for the young people in prisons and for my patients would never compensate for the pain and confusion I would cause them. I was a source of inspiration to them; my death would take everything away from them.

All my life, when painful or difficult times arose, I would think of death, but never before did I consider it the way I did at that time. For days, I would get in the car and drive. I had just begun to use my car as my main means of transportation. I didn't know the roads well so I just went onto the main freeway and drove straight along the ocean, along the mountain, from early morning until late afternoon, and then I would turn around and drive back.

Many times as I was driving by the mountainside, I felt impelled to plunge my car downwards. It would just take one movement. My hand would swerve and the car would go. I could not do it, however—not because I wanted to live so badly but because I could not bear thinking about the pain that I would cause the people who would still be alive, especially my own brother.

So the only other alternative was to go to Plum Village Monastery. I had met our Teacher, Thay, three weeks before, and I had faith in him and in the Dharma. Deep inside me, besides the despair, there was a deep faith and confidence that I could find true peace within myself.

ESCAPING DEATH TWICE

About two weeks after John's death and before I went to Plum Village, I drove to the hospital where I was working to return some books and to say good-bye to the director of the program and my fellow residents. The director kindly said to me that if I wanted, he would keep the position open for me for five years, so I could take time off to care for myself. I thanked him and told him that I didn't want to make any contract or any promise. I just wanted to find peace.

After I said good-bye to them, I began to drive toward Hayward to attend a ceremony for my partner John. Venerable Tu Luc was living in Hayward, and he was helping me conduct weekly ceremonies for John until the forty-ninth day after his passing.

As I was driving on the freeway, a woman in the car in front of me put out her hand, pointing to my car, and when she finally caught my attention, I realized that the front of my car was smoking. I immediately took the next exit and as a normal reaction, I put my foot on the brake to slow down. To my complete surprise, the car didn't slow down. I pressed harder on the brakes, but it still kept going. Even when I pressed down completely on the brakes, the car went on as if there were no brakes at all. It was flying down the exit ramp at full speed.

In that moment, images came to my mind. It was like a movie fast-forwarded. In my mind screen, images of my life surfaced like snapshots. Something in me knew exactly what each of those snapshots meant. There was no need to use my intellectual mind to understand them. Each snapshot flashed by quickly and there was a deep sense of knowing that it was a review of my entire life. All those moments flashed by, and I simply watched them.

The only thought I had this whole time was that John had died a beautiful death, but I was going to die a violent death. Besides that one thought, I didn't feel any kind of anxiety or fear. I just continued to hold on to the wheel. My car came off the exit, went into the city and drove past green lights and red lights until it had no more momentum, and then it just stopped dead on a large street with hardly anyone on it.

I got out of the car. It was still smoking. I tried to open the hood, but it was too hot, so I left the car there and walked quite a distance to the nearest store. I knew little about cars, and my logic was that it was burning, and I needed to pour water on it to cool it off.

I bought three big bottles of water, but then I realized I could not carry them because they were heavy, and my car was far away. I saw an impressively large man by the checkout counter, and I asked him, "My car broke down and I need to pour water on it. Would you help me to transport this water?"

He looked at me and he said, "Sure, I can drive you." So I got in his truck, a big four-wheel-drive, and he drove me to the car. He took a look at the situation and said, "I think something is wrong with the cooling system. You cannot pour water on it. It would just crack it."

I asked him to help me find a place that could fix my car. Then I proceeded to tell him about my dilemma, that I needed to go to this ceremony for my partner who just passed away a few weeks ago, and that I needed to take care of this car.

He agreed, drove me to a car dealer and talked to them for me. I could leave my car there on the street, and they promised they would come to tow it away and fix it. Then I asked him to drive me to the train station, and again, he was willing to help me.

While he was driving, I started to ask about him and his family situation. He told me that he was a Harley Davidson rider and that was his hobby. He had a daughter, but he and his wife were divorced. His daughter was a teenager and he was quite worried about her because he didn't have good communication at all with her or with his former wife.

Being the young doctor and the friendly person that I was, I offered him a lot of advice. He was overweight, so I told him that he needed to exercise in order to have good health and to be there for his daughter. I encouraged him to try to keep in touch with her because she needed a father. I hadn't had a father as I was growing up and it was a major part of my life that was missing, so I hoped he could be there for his daughter.

We talked at length. I also told him about my partner and how he died. Somewhere along the way, I began to notice that we had been driving for a long time. Then I saw we were driving into the desert, further and further until there were no cars at all. He took a turn onto a dirt trail, and at that time, I became silent. I didn't ask him where he was driving me. Something in me sensed that I was in a dangerous situation.

I remained silent. I began to see occasional trailers. The whole place was dilapidated—neither cared for, nor inhabited. He finally stopped in front of one trailer. It felt spooky.

He said, "I need to make a phone call before we go." I didn't say anything and just sat in the truck. He went into his trailer and stayed in there for what seemed a long time. I assessed my situation. I knew I couldn't run away because it was in the middle of nowhere, and he had taken the key with him and put it in his pocket. There was no way I could run and no way I could scream for help, so I opened the truck door and got out.

I stepped up the stairs to his trailer, and then one step past the threshold. I saw him. The trailer was dark, not well kept and not decorated with anything. There was a bed. Next to it was a table, and he was standing there. He looked up at me. I could feel his hesitation. He looked down. I stepped backward, out of the threshold, very slowly down the steps, and back to his truck where I stood by the door.

I just stood there. I don't know how long it went on, but it seemed like eternity. He finally came out, got in the truck and said, "Let's go." I still remember the hard, dry sound of his door being slammed shut. I got into the truck and we drove away.

This time, we never said another word to each other during the whole drive. When we got to the train station, I said to him, "I owe you my life. I'm deeply grateful to you." I opened my arms and hugged him. He was a gigantic man. I didn't stand taller than his armpit, and my arms could not circle all the way around him, but I hugged him with all of my sincere might.

Then I got on the train to get to the temple in time for John's ceremony. I realized I had been in near-death situations twice that day. The first time was when my car lost its brakes on the freeway, but that death wouldn't have been as violent and as painful as the second death that I might have faced with this man.

He would have hurt me, and he most likely would have killed me. I only recognized that much and I didn't have a chance to process that experience further because there were many visits to make and many other things to take care of before I went to Plum Village in France.

As I became more settled in Plum Village, memories about that day arose strongly. I realized that what saved me was that somehow I saw the situation and I could accept it. I was not panicking in either situation. I could simply be with what was unfolding.

I also saw that I had treated the man as a human being. I didn't have any kind of judgment toward him, even though I knew he drove a Harley Davidson motorcycle, and there's this stereotype that they are rough people, but my heart was open and kind to him as my fellow human being. I was concerned about his health, about his family, and about his happiness. We talked to each other at a real level, and I truly believe it touched the human seed in him and the Buddha seed in him.

So even though the seeds of craving and ruthlessness in him came up—maybe he had done that to other women before—and he was about to do that to me, he didn't have the heart. He hesitated. All that was needed was a moment of hesitation, and then he could not do it. During that whole time, I didn't try to run. I didn't try to scream. I didn't say anything that was fearful or hateful. In those moments, I actually remained calm and quiet in my own mind, and that helped not to provoke violence or trigger more excitement in him.

The appropriate response may be different depending on the situation. In the life-threatening situations I have been in, I've learned that staying calm is the most powerful thing I can do.

BEAUTIFUL DANCE

John's life made me look at death more closely. The only way I could accept his death was to learn to accept my own death. I learn that I am dying during my daily life.

When I first became a nun, I cried a lot, and Thay would help me in several ways. One time while we were standing at the check-in point of the airport, watching our luggage going through the machine, Thay gently said to me, "You see that luggage? It comes in this side, and it goes out on the other side. Birth and death are also like that."

It was simple the way Thay said it, but to this day I remember, "It comes in this side, and it goes out on the other side."

Another time at the airport, I was there to see Thay going off to the

United States for the teaching tour in 2001. He had already checked in and was standing on the other side of a glass door. He waved at me, and when I came close to him, he said through the crevice between two glass panels, "My child, stay home and practice walking meditation."

Another time, Thay said to me, "My child, the cats and the dogs are also your *su em*; they need your help too." "Su" means teacher and "em" means younger brother or younger sister. So the dogs and cats are my teachers as well as my younger siblings. In this way, Thay would teach me about death, about the value of life that I needed to nurture and to care for, so that every time the thought of suicide or death arose in my mind, I slowly learned to say to myself, "Death is happening. It is taking place. I don't have to wish for it." I see the value and connection of my own life to other living beings, including the animals.

When I wish for death, my mind is discriminating between birth and death. Mindfulness helps me to see that birth and death are taking place in every moment. I live and die every moment. Birth and death are like a beautiful dance—one step forward, one step backward, no coming, no going, spinning, twirling. . . .

When I think an unskillful thought, it kills something inside me. It causes a death in me, and it causes a death in somebody else.

On the other hand, if I think of something nurturing, that can bring life to me, and it can inspire life in someone else.

In my spiritual practice, I am blessed to acknowledge death and birth and their interbeing nature. It is not only at the last breath that I touch death, but I am able to touch it at every moment, and I have a choice to live or to die at every moment.

It is empowering to know that I have the power to affect how I die and how I live in every moment. I can live deeply each moment, so I can be free from the habit of grasping either life or death and avoiding the other.

I talked to a woman whose boyfriend had died when she was seventeen. She was already in her early forties, but when she recounted her boyfriend's death, it was as if it had just happened that morning. Her pain was still unbearable. Ever since his death, she could not have a normal relationship with anyone else.

As I looked at her, I asked myself, "Do I want to become like this woman?" In my old age, all I would have accumulated were losses and suffering. I didn't want that. I wanted to choose peace.

Thus, I practice to live in the present moment. This has taught me that when your loved one has died, and you are drowning in suffering and forgetting to live your life, then your loved one is truly dead, nothing but a ghost of the past. Every time you think about that person when he or she was alive, the memories pain you and kill you slowly. In this way, you are actually making sure that your beloved is as dead as he or she can be, as you are wasting your own life away.

On the contrary, if you live your life fully and meaningfully, then you see your beloved in everything you do and in everything you see. You allow him or her the chance to grow with you and to live on.

John loved the color purple. Every time I see purple flowers I think of him. He loved nature, and as a nun, I have more time and opportunity to be in nature. I have learned to care for myself the way John cared for me;

his hands have become my own hands, and his hands are now the hands of my monastic sisters and brothers.

When I hear birds making cuckoo sounds, I stop to smile and listen, because that was what John used to do to call for my attention. Awareness of the wonders of life allows you to see your beloved in everything. You are no longer caught in that particular form that has now disintegrated into the earth or into the water. You see new manifestations everywhere, and these help you to celebrate life and feel deeply connected, not to just one person, but to all that is.

John has become me, he is me, and I live this life for him. There is no separation between us anymore. Before I go to sleep, I can say to myself, "If tonight I do not wake up, I have no regret."

OCEAN AND WAVE

I will tell you a story
About the wave and the ocean.
Since an unknown time
The wave feels all alone.
She searches for the ocean
In endless outward directions.

The wave is full of desires,
And the ocean is vast.
The wave keeps on looking,
But the ocean is still far, far away.

There are nights by the gentle moon
The wave holds herself in stillness.
Suddenly she feels immense.
The ocean whispers inside her.

At times she is howling,
Raging in rapid successions,
Indulging in self-destruction,
Because ignorance from infinite time
Would not want to rest.

Only the wave understands
How vast the ocean is.
Only the ocean knows
Where the wave goes and returns to.

Those days when the wave vagabonds,
The ocean patiently awaits.
Those days when the wave plunges into despair,
The ocean continues to embrace.

If the wave sees the ocean
She would no longer need to search.

If you know that we are in each other
You will fear no more.

—December 2003

Chapter Seven

ONENESS

SPANNING A BRIDGE

This is the story of my personal experience during our Teacher's return to Vietnam in 2007. In the southern, central, and northern regions of the country, Thay conducted a series of ceremonies, known as the Great Requiem Ceremonies to Pray Equally for All People and to Untie the Knots of Injustices, thus creating favorable conditions for his disciples and his people to uproot and remove deep internal formations and suffering from the Vietnam War. During this trip I returned to visit Quang Ngai, the place of my birth, for the first time since I had left it at the age of six.

FOR LOVE TO DEEPEN

My chest felt like a heavy cement block. My in-breath and out-breath were superficial and laborious. I intentionally forced my abdomen to rise and fall, but oxygen seemed not to have enough space to enter the lower part of the lungs. I had assisted in surgical procedures that were eight to ten hours long, which had caused me to have back and abdominal pain, but I never experienced chest discomfort like this.

I relaxed my shoulders and arms, and I continued to follow my breathing. The powerful chanting of the monks stirred my deep consciousness. I saw thousands of skeleton figures standing on the water and coming toward the shore without moving. The immense ocean was without waves. Everything about those skeletons and the space around them was gray and foggy. Suddenly, I realized that I had seen these images fifteen years before, when I was still a medical student at the University of California, San Francisco, School of Medicine. There were afternoons when I had wandered aimlessly along the beach. I had stood watching those gray skeleton figures, not knowing how they were related to me and to the pervasive sadness always haunting me. I wrote about them at that time in a poem, titled "Dreams":

> These days my limbs guide me near the waters.
> The sky is gray.
> Still, the waves are grayer.
> I see stick figures through the mist.
> Forever claimed by the sea,
> They walk without moving.
> Something whispers:
> "Walk straight. Walk straight."
> My heart pulsates, but I am drawn to silence.

Now, I also saw people falling down in an open field; I saw little children screaming wide-mouthed and lying exhausted on their mothers' corpses; I saw a naked woman curling up in a bush; I saw layers of people stacked on each other. I saw. I saw so much . . .

I continued to follow my breathing. I hadn't known that these images and the innumerable possible deaths were stored in my consciousness! Everything I had ever seen, heard, and perceived; everything my parents, ancestors, and society had ever seen, heard, and perceived—they all had been imprinted in my mind! Tears streamed down. Sweat oozed from me in big droplets, even from places I hadn't known could perspire. My whole body seemed to be excreting . . . and purifying.

I stood still . . . so that the young girl in my mother could be absolved from injustices. That young girl had left her arid homeland in Quang Ngai to go to work in Saigon. She became a maid, and she saved every penny to send home to her mother, my grandmother. Each night, the owner came to her little corner at the back of the house. She curled up under her bamboo bed, but he wouldn't let her be. He used a broom to poke her and get her out. The young girl wandered on the street. Her education was minimal. She had no skills, and circumstances pushed her as it had pushed countless young girls in war time. She worked for American soldiers, and she gave birth to my brother and me—two more Amerasian children who didn't know their fathers' faces or names. Then, my mother became a mistress of a rich old man, only for the purpose of taking care of her children and her relatives. There were times when my mother would yell at me and beat me up as if I were her enemy. Afterward, while I was sleeping, she would rub green oil on my bruises and cry. She only thought about getting away; her dream was to go to America. On the fifth of May in 1980, my mother went to the market for work as usual, but she never came back. She disappeared at the age of thirty-six. I was only twelve then. I remember squatting on the toilet seat, thinking, "Good, from now on she will not abuse me anymore!"

I stood still . . . so the father inside my brother could be absolved from injustices. My brother was born with blond hair and fair skin. He was so beautiful that I wrapped an embroidered tablecloth around his face and his body; he looked like a princess, and I carried him on my hip everywhere. Yet children in the neighborhood kept calling him "Amerasian with twelve butt holes!" They spit on him. They made him the American prisoner in their war games. My grandmother was well aware that if my brother remained in Vietnam, he would be teased and shamed and exploited his whole life. Nevertheless, sending him to the United States was like severing her own intestines. Ironically, when he did get to the United States, children in his American school shouted at him, "Communist, go home!" because he didn't speak any English. Like a wounded animal, my brother lashed out in fury and beat up those kids with all his might. The psychologist diagnosed him as having "extreme uncontrolled anger." The United States government paid money to put my brother in a rehabilitation center for rich kids who had problems with drug addiction, gangs, and violence. My brother was now thirty-five years old, built like a football player. In his house, there are over sixty guns of different sizes; stacks of bullets lie all over. He is a licensed gun dealer. In his house, there are over a hundred videos about the Vietnam War and other violent crimes. My brother can't sleep without the television on all night. His eyes are gentle and bright, and he smiles often. Yet, my brother's mind has a dark side, which continues to damage and push him.

I stood still . . . so my uncles could be absolved from injustices. My oldest uncle, Uncle Number Two, ran away from home to the North to become a Communist. Every so often, soldiers of the South Vietnam Republic would call my grandmother to their post, to beat her and harass her about my uncle. After the defeat of the South Vietnam Republic by the Communists in 1975, my uncle came south to Saigon to look for his mother and siblings. He brought with him a white pillowcase with red words, "Returning to Motherland" on it. He had embroidered it while serving on the Ho Chi Minh Trail. My uncle enthusiastically took my grandmother to the North to meet his wife and three children. However, he died within six months. Years of suffering from malnutrition, bouts of malaria, tons of bombs and chemical warfare had damaged his heart, lungs, liver, and intestines. My grandmother returned to the South alone, too stunned to cry.

My youngest uncle, Uncle Number Six, ran away from our home in Quang Ngai to look for my mother in Saigon when he was thirteen years old. Not being able to find my mother at first, he lived on the streets, polished shoes, stole things, got involved in reckless sexual activity, and later joined the army of the Republic of South Vietnam. After the defeat of the south by the Communists, my mother sent him to a distant farmland, so he could avoid the Communist rehabilitation camp. He got involved in drinking and womanizing again. His neighbors got angry and turned him in to the police. My uncle escaped from prison by swimming more than twenty-five kilometers along the river, but once he got close to our house, he sent word to fetch my grandmother. He didn't dare to come into the house, because he feared my mother! I remember when my uncle got drunk, he was quite jolly, but my mother became incensed. Once, he crawled under the bed, and my mother was still hitting him with a broom. My uncle slurred, "Wide-mouth big sister, please forgive your little brother." My uncle died before he turned fifty-five years old. Cigarettes, liquor, and women had drained all of his life energy.

I stood still . . . so the Vows to the Dead and the compassionate energy of the Three Jewels—the Buddha, the Dharma, and the Sangha—could absolve all injustices for my people, those with names but bodies never found, those with bodies but names untraceable, those who died because of injustice, those who lived in repression, those who continued to be choked and repressed inside our own consciousness, whether we were aware of them or not.

Sometimes we can only breathe at the neck or chest level, when our body is tense and restless, or we feel stressed and agitated. We don't understand why we think, speak, and behave so negatively and cynically. That is because the undercurrents of suffering from countless generations, although invisible, nevertheless continue to ravage our lives. Recognizing these forces and calling them by their true names is to span a bridge into the depth of our store consciousness, so that the dead inside the living can dwell with lightness, so that the living who hold the dead within can truly live.

Tears streamed down my face, but I did not suffer.

After the second night of the ceremony, I felt lighter and I could breathe normally again. A young brother said to me, "I saw you crying. I really wanted to bring my handkerchief to you, to wipe your tears, but when I pulled it out of my pocket, it looked black with sweat!"

Those days of March 2007 were scorching, but people came to participate in the ceremony from early morning to late evening. Seven thousand, then ten thousand food portions were still not enough to provide for everyone. One woman said she stayed for the ceremony even until it was very late "because ceremonies like this only happen once every hundred years." Another woman corrected her, "It won't happen again for another thousand years!"

I gave thanks to Thay, who had been able to untie the knots inside himself, so that he could establish the Requiem Ceremonies to Pray Equally for All People and to Untie the Knots of Injustices in them, creating favorable conditions for his disciples and his people to uproot and remove deep internal formations.

Someone cried and asked, "Who is this Grandfather Monk, who loves us and our deceased so much?"

Each day, when a ceremony was beginning, the monastic Sangha would do walking meditation from outside the Ancestors' Hall, to the front court, then to the main hall of Temple Vinh Nghiem Pagoda (Adornment with Eternity) in Saigon.

Sixty young monks from Prajna Temple (Bat Nha Monastery in the Central Highlands of Vietnam) walked in front, holding up ceremonial instruments, followed by the Chanting Master of Ceremonies (Venerable Le Trang), Thay, the assisting chanting monks, the musicians, the high venerables, and over two hundred monks and nuns from Plum Village, Prajna, and Tu Hieu (Thay's root temple outside Hue). Thousands of people watched the procession in complete silence and respect.

Most ceremonies took place in the main hall, and laypeople could only observe them by looking in from outside or by watching two big screens in the courtyard. Still, everyone participated wholeheartedly and offered up their concentrated energies to the dead souls.

Some people had wondered why Thay, a Zen master, would have these ceremonies performed in the Vajrayana (Tantric) tradition. Suddenly, I appreciated the wonderful meaning of "skillful means." It's certain that thousands of beginners, like me, wouldn't be able to meditate and concentrate their minds continuously for three days, but they could more easily follow these Tantric ceremonies and benefit from them.

Venerable Le Trang and his co-chanters understood Thay's deepest wish. They gave their whole bodies and minds to the Requiem Ceremony, so that it attained the highest success. Later, when Thay and the delegation were about to leave for Hong Kong, Venerable Le Trang and his co-chanters flew to Hanoi to personally say farewell to Thay one more time. All of our brothers and sisters were moved by their deep love. Thay looked happy, and the Venerable Le Trang's face also radiated pure joy. Sitting next to him, Thay said, "On this trip, we have met soul mates, like Venerable Le Trang and his brothers. Because the Great Requiem Ceremony in Vinh Nghiem succeeded, the Great Requiem Ceremony in Dieu De succeeded, and because the Great Requiem Ceremony in Dieu De succeeded, the Great Requiem Ceremony in Soc Son was completed successfully."

The Vietnamese origin legend tells the tale of a Mother who came from the heaven and a Father who came from the sea. Their union gave birth to one hundred children, fifty of whom went back to the sea with the father and fifty of whom remained on land with the mother. Their descendents are forever brothers and sisters. True to the spirit of this legend, the Chanting Masters worked to bring together people from the southern, central, and northern parts of Vietnam. Christians and Buddhists came together for these historic moments.

STILL WITH FAITH

When my bus arrived at Tu Hieu Temple, in Hue in Central Vietnam, Thay and the Sangha were visiting at nearby Tu Dam Temple. A group of monastics from Prajna had arrived a few days before. A sister told us to put on our sanghatis and prepare to greet Thay at Tu Hieu.

I didn't feel well, so I rested at Dieu Nghiem. When the sisters came back, an elder sister said, "It's just us greeting each other. The early arrivals greet the late arrivals." That was a lot of fun!

During the time that Thay and the delegation were in Hue, the number of people coming to visit and participate in retreats was much less than when Thay returned the first time in 2005. I didn't feel discouraged by the change in people's hearts. Those moments shared together two years earlier—the joyful smiles and the trusting eyes—were real, and they will continue to be beautiful in my heart.

The activities continued to take place as planned. Thay gave Dharma talks with utmost compassion and inclusiveness. Sometimes while I was translating into English, I felt so dizzy and nauseated. I looked at Thay. He sat stably, and his eyes were penetrating. I thought, "I love you so much, Thay. You are incredibly courageous!" My mind could concentrate again. I listened and translated Thay's talk from Vietnamese to English for the two hundred international lay friends who were part of the Plum Village delegation.

The monastic Sangha sat together for two days before the Great Requiem Ceremony began in Hue. Brother Phap An shared with the Sangha the many difficulties he and the pioneering team had encountered as they prepared for the ceremonies. Unlike our experience in Saigon, the support from the Buddhist Church and the government in Hue was unreliable. Brother Phap An emphasized that the support in Hanoi was even more fragile.

Our Sangha was responsible for everything from A to Z. Brother Phap An wanted the younger brothers and sisters to be aware of the situation, so that we would contribute wholeheartedly our practice and our service. I was deeply grateful to Brother Phap An, our preparation team, and all brothers and sisters from Prajna and Tu Hieu. Everybody worked tirelessly day and night, transcending their own physical and mental limitations.

The success of each Requiem Ceremony in the southern, central, and northern regions of Vietnam wasn't due to any one individual or organization. Innumerable hands, minds, and hearts joined together to make history. The peoples' hearts wanted it; the collective consciousness had ripened. While there was some dissension within the party, a few important government officials made key interventions that enabled Thay's presence in Vietnam and the Requiem Ceremonies possible. Just as it was during the war, Thay's attempts to bring the people together was viewed as highly political, controversial, and threatening to many Vietnamese communist officials, to the Chinese government, and even to a number of Vietnamese Buddhist monastic leaders. Thus, even though there were forces opposing it, there was nothing that could stop it.

The Requiem Ceremony was to be held at Temple Dieu De (Wonderful Truth) in Hue, which had a river flowing peacefully in front of it. Many children and elderly people begged at the gate. The temple was small, so all the altars—for the souls of the dead, for Kshitigarbha Bodhisattva, for Amitabha Buddha, as well as Kshitigarbha's lion throne—were set up, in that order, from near the gate to the front of the Buddha Hall.

The Great Requiem Ceremony began with the Invitation of Masters. About five Most Venerables came to offer their witness to this important opening. Even though they were old and their disciples had to help them walk, they still exuded powerful spiritual strength from many generations.

Thay wore the ceremonial sanghati that he had worn in Vinh Nghiem. I remember the first time Thay appeared in that stately robe—heavy and large and it veiled his whole body—he looked like the Bodhisattva

Avalokiteshvara. Tears streamed down my cheeks. Thay usually wore his brown robe and brown Tiep Hien jacket for Order of Interbeing members. He didn't like cumbersome ceremonies or fancy outfits. Because of us, he went through all of this! (Later in Thailand, at the praying ceremony for King Rama IX's long life, all the monastics from over fifty countries wore their ceremonial sanghatis, except for Thay; he wore his brown robe and brown Tiep Hien jacket. Seeing that deepened my appreciation for the choice he made at Temple Dieu De.)

After the Invitation of the Masters ceremony, a number of monastics and Order of Interbeing members followed Thay, the Chanting Master and his co-chanters to go invite the spirits to come back to Temple Dieu De, in order to receive food offerings and Dharma offerings during the next three days.

On a mountain near the temple, Mount Ban, a bamboo pole was put up with a long length of white cloth, which symbolized a bridge that those who had died on land could walk on to follow us back to the temple. At a river, another length of white cloth was lowered into the water, so that those who had died in the water could climb onto dry land and follow us back to the temple.

The heat of the day was unbearable. Sweat dripped profusely. Some local young people were smoking and chatting nearby. I said to them softly, "The monks and nuns are praying for the people who died in the Vietnam War. Certainly this includes many of your relatives. You could contribute your part and pray for them." One-by-one, they extinguished their cigarettes and stood quietly for the rest of the ceremony.

There was also a funeral procession passing by on a small boat, for a child who had fallen into the water the day before. Probably her family lived on that boat. The mother looked disheveled. I prayed for the child and for her family.

After the Invitation of the Souls of the Dead ceremony was completed, the two lengths of white cloth were hung at the gate of the temple. A food offering ceremony was performed. Monks and nuns from the Buddhist Institute also came to recite the sutra about Kshitigarbha Bodhisattva. Over two thousand people attended the first day of the Requiem Ceremony in Hue. They stood along both sides of the Buddha Hall to observe all the ceremonies. The heat was extreme. Water could not be supplied in a sufficient amount.

In the late afternoon, I went for a walk along the river with a younger sister. A well-dressed gentleman on his scooter stopped me to ask, "What is the name of the police officer who spoke at Hue Festival Centre last night?"

I answered enthusiastically, "Her name is Cheri." He took out a notebook and asked me to spell her name. A thought crossed my mind that he might be up to something negative, so I didn't spell her last name to him. Once he got her name, he sped away. My sister told me, "He's probably an undercover cop. He wants to investigate whether she's truly a police officer in the United States."

Cheri had spoken only about ten minutes at Thay's Dharma talk at Hue Festival Centre but, in fact, she had also written a six-page report to inform Thay about everything she had been able to do for her police department, the prisons, and the young people's court in Wisconsin and in other states. She had applied the Buddhist teachings and practices learned at Plum Village to her work and home. With the experiences and insights gained from her own practice, she used her political influence to bring positive and creative changes. I remembered that she used to have the tough look of police officers when I first met her at Plum Village and at the retreat in Wisconsin; now she looked light and humble. Her gaze and her words reflected deep respect and love for Thay, as well as for Vietnam, where her spiritual roots are.

The presence of Cheri Maples, and of hundreds of Western lay practitioners and monastics of the Plum Village International Sangha, spanned a bridge into the hearts of the Vietnamese people, transforming many long-term, ingrained perceptions. If, perhaps, to Vietnamese people, Westerners represent an invading force, they also represent a prosperous civilization. Perhaps Vietnamese people very much wish to participate in the globalization movement, but in the depths of their consciousness, they may still bear hatred and suspicion toward Westerners.

Looking at the Western monks, nuns, and lay friends standing and touching the Earth so solemnly during the many ceremonies, which went on from four to eight hours, many Vietnamese people were deeply moved. One French sister was present at every ceremony, even though she was over sixty years old. She shared with me, "I regret and feel ashamed, because my ancestors caused a lot of suffering to the land and the people of Vietnam. I want to kneel with my monastic sisters and brothers during the ceremony in order to apologize for my ancestors."

It rained hard that night. Then, it drizzled the whole next day and made the air cool and pleasant. On the second night, there was a ceremony to open the gates of hell and to transmit the Three Refugees and Five Mindfulness Trainings to the souls of the dead. Following is the deep sharing by Sister Truc Nghiem, also known as Sister Bamboo, about this ceremony:

It was raining, but not heavily. It drizzled enough to soak the streets, people's clothes, and my own heart. It cried for Hue, for the people who are still deep in poverty. The elderly mothers and grandmothers in their stiffened, old shirts, their arms and legs dry and thin like sticks, curling up in front of the temple or trembling as they begged for food. The images, recounted by sister Nhu Minh, about hundreds of people buried alive . . . then bombing . . . then a flood . . . were still shaking me.

The Chanting Master of the ceremony, representing Kshitigarbha Bodhisattva, recited mantras in order to open the gates of hell. He recited Plum Village's version of The Heart of Perfect Understanding in Hue's musical style; his voice was sweet and sincere, expressing empathy and the wish for all victims in the dark realms to take refuge in the energy of the Three Jewels, in order to come to the ceremony, to listen to the Dharma, and to receive the Five Mindfulness Trainings.

He dropped a big roll of white cloth, which spanned a bridge from hell to Earth. The roll of cloth began to unroll. No one said anything, but suddenly, the grandmothers, the mothers, uncles, aunts, young and old, men and women, all rushed in to carry the cloth above their heads. Hundreds of people were making a cloth bridge. Those who could not get in reached out their hands to hold on to the edge of the cloth bridge or to hold on to the shirt of those holding it up. Head to head, shoulder to shoulder, everyone in the world of the living was working together to span a bridge for those in the world of the dead. The cloth bridge had no limit, and the worlds of the living and of the dead also had no boundary!

Suddenly, I understood the meaning of, 'The memorial white cloth for Hue.' Regardless of all losses and suffering endured by Hue, there's always something harmonizing between life and death. I know it's Love that opens the gateway to these two worlds and helps them bear the suffering together.

The most significant part of the Great Requiem Ceremony took place on the very last night. It was called the "Chan Te" (Helping to Cross Over) ceremony, which helped the dead souls to do Beginning Anew for their past wrong actions, to transform their suffering, and to aspire for complete liberation.

The Chanting Master ascended the lion throne of Kshitigarbha Bodhisattva, and the co-chanters sat on both sides in front of the lion throne. The monastics sat behind the co-chanters. Thousands of laypeople arranged themselves all around us. Those who were far away stood on chairs. The whole temple ground was packed. In that solemn atmosphere, I nevertheless also felt the coziness of a big family sitting around each other.

There was one chanted phrase that affected me deeply: "Not knowing that you have lost your own body, your mind is unclear, confused, uncertain where it is going." I thought of the people on heroin, lying listlessly in a dark space, their bodies going limp, their consciousness becoming clouded, not in touch with their own bodies, not aware of their mind states. How many of us are living like sleepwalkers? How many hungry ghosts are wandering in our civilized society?

The Chanting Master recited The Ten Kinds of Hungry Ghosts. After each kind of ghost, the co-chanting monks simultaneously recited mantras to untie the internal knots for them. They had become hungry ghosts because they had died in battles; while running away from invaders; while giving birth (both mothers and children); while serving as concubines or dancers in royal palaces; while being sold for their bodies; while feeling in despair and taking their own lives—these victims became hungry ghosts. Their suffering and injustices continued to dwell in the deep layers of consciousness of their loved ones and of society.

The Chanting Master threw a handful of rice over the audience. People in that direction leaned forward to catch it. Everyone wanted to receive some of this rice, because it was empowered by the energy of the Three Jewels. They would save it and use it for treating various ailments.

Each fifty-kilogram sack of rice was poured onto the table of the Chanting Master. He then recited mantras and did *mudra* hand gestures over the rice to bless it. Then the assisting monks would scoop up the rice in small bowls and cups to distribute it to the people.

The more rice that was distributed, the more people squeezed in to receive it. Some monastic sisters next to me had already left, so there was empty space all around me. The people were closing in, right up to my neck, but because I sat solidly, they didn't dare to pass by me. Finally, I felt that their energy was becoming too strong, so I unfolded my legs and stood up.

Within a split-second, everyone behind me poured forward. The waves of people were about to engulf and overturn everything. All the monastic brothers and sisters immediately stood up, stretched out our arms sideways, and held each other's hands to create a wall of yellow sanghati robes surrounding and protecting the Chanting Master and the co-chanters, so that they could continue with the ceremony.

I saw a number of Western monastics standing on the opposite side of the circle; they were holding the ceremonial poles with one hand and holding on to the next monastic with the other hand. The human waves continued to push forward. Hundreds, then thousands of hands were reaching out to beg for rice. Many were raising up plastic bags or funnels made of paper.

Some people's eyes looked so sincere. There were also eyes filled with deep thirst and hunger; their owners shoved everyone, including the monastics, crudely and violently. The monastics were holding back the human waves with our own bodies, and, at the same time, distributing rice to them. Each time, as I gave out a handful of rice, I breathed in and placed my folded hand in that person's palm; then I breathed out and released the rice into his or her palm. That moment of contact was sacred, and I felt the thirst and hunger within that person was instantaneously satisfied.

The Chan Te ceremony was completed successfully. Everyone dispersed quickly. An Israeli sister recounted that because the Western sisters were still holding up the ceremonial poles in their hands, they followed Brother Phap An to walk the Chanting Master and the co-chanting monks back to Temple Ong, right next to Temple Dieu De. Inside the Buddha Hall, Brother Phap An asked permission to touch the Earth to express our deep gratitude to the Chanting Masters. The Chanting Masters refused to accept the prostrations and began to remove their sanghati robes. Brother Phap An nevertheless knelt down and touched the Earth deeply. The sisters were standing at the threshold outside the Buddha Hall, where shoes were left and the ground was muddy, but because they also wanted to express their gratitude, they, too, touched the Earth deeply right where they were.

CLEARING THE STREAM

Once again, the Sangha packed up, this time to go to Da Nang and Nha Trang, before we continued on to Hanoi.

During our time in Da Nang, I went to visit my birthplace, Quang Ngai, after being away for thirty-three years. I had been back to Vietnam three times, all before I ordained, but I'd never had the desire to return to Quang Ngai. This time, I came home, and I believe that the Great Requiem Ceremonies in southern and central Vietnam had cleared the ancestral stream in me.

I walked slowly on the road that I used to walk on to my elementary school. The bamboo bridge was no longer there; the streambed had been filled up flat and a sewage tunnel ran underneath it.

I was born during the 1968 Tet Offensive, and my homeland was severely bombed. Houses were destroyed, so my whole family had to run away. When I was less than a week old, two men carried my mother away on a hammock, and my auntie was running in front with me in her arms. My grandmother said that they should separate my mother and me so that if a bomb hit us we wouldn't both die. They carried us a long way, but no one in the adjacent village wanted to house my mother and me, because it was believed that a woman who had recently given birth carried very negative energy that would bring extremely bad luck to the host.

In the end, a cousin of my mother agreed to bring us into his home.

Now, when he heard that I had come back to visit, he rode a bicycle to come to see me. He was in his seventies now, wearing a black hat and a black outfit. His features were handsome and elegant. I kept staring at him during the whole visit, and my tears kept streaming down.

He exclaimed, "Lo and behold, she looks just like that little girl Number Five!" My mother had been the fifth in her family.

I asked him, "Why did you take us in, when everyone was afraid of bad luck, of becoming poor for the rest of their lives?"

He replied, "I thought, she is my cousin. If I don't help her, who will? After you came to stay with us, my wife became very sick for many years, and it was true that we were poor for our whole lives. I never believed it was because of you and your mother. Being poor is a part of my destiny, that's all. What is most important is that I offer love and kindness to others from the beginning to the end."

He continued, "I made a little bamboo hut for your mother and you behind my house. There was a bamboo grove in the garden, so I dug a deep hole in its shade and placed a log over it, so your mother could relieve herself discreetly. I still remember the neighbor looking over from his house, shaking his head, as he said, 'Young Brother Number Six, you just involve yourself in futile work!' I disregarded the remarks people made."

He had continued to live in that simple house with his wife. I asked permission to visit the backyard. My mother's hut was now just a barren spot; the bamboo grove had recently been cut down and the bamboo branches were still lying on the ground! Before I left, I ransacked my brown bag: Ensure in a plastic bag, forty-some Vitamin C tablets, half a bottle of green oil, and a stack of Band-Aids. I asked my uncle to accept them for me. I gave my auntie all the money I had, so that she could help him get a complete set of dentures made. "When you eat and you can chew vegetables easily, think of me," I told him.

HANDS OF FLOWER

Temple Non (Temple Mountain) was situated in a secluded area near Hanoi in northern Vietnam. It seemed that there were no dwellings in the vicinity within three or four kilometers. The mountain road leading to Temple Non was long, steep, and deserted.

The Buddhist Institute of Soc Son was about halfway up the mountain road, and the temple was at the end, snuggled entirely inside the U-shaped valley of the mountain. Besides the Buddha Hall, there was only a flat building with about five rooms and one public toilet—and that was everything!

Thay gave two Dharma talks to the young monks and nuns from the Buddhist Institute before the Great Requiem Ceremony began at Temple Non. Only about fifty of them came. They sat inside the Buddha Hall in the corner with our Western monastics, and that almost filled up the hall already. The rest sat on the veranda. The decorations inside and outside the main hall seemed to be as they usually were, and there was no visible sign that the Great Requiem Ceremony would be starting in two days.

The brothers from Prajna were still carrying banners and flags up and down the mountain road, looking for places to hang them up. I heard whispers saying, "The temple is too far away. Probably there'll be just us for this ceremony. We have to try to attend all the ceremonies and send our energies wholeheartedly."

To our utmost astonishment, on the morning of the ceremony, many small vendors sprouted up on both sides of the mountain road, as if they had come from under the Earth. Hundreds of big vans and small vans parked at the bottom of the road as well as in the parking lot across from the Buddhist Institute. Thousands of people, old and young, men and women, enthusiastically climbed the slope. Someone said, "I heard the monks and nuns will have a great ceremony for us, so I came."

Amplifiers were set up on the veranda and along the road, so that people could sit wherever they could find a place and listen to all the ceremonies. People in the northern region had a tradition of burning excessive amounts of paper money, paper clothes, and so forth for the dead to use. I heard a monk with a northern accent making the announcement, "Please, we ask everyone not to burn paper money. We have many people here, and we need to protect the environment and our health. Please do not burn paper money during the next three days of the ceremony."

The veranda of the temple had transformed completely. The Altar of Amitabha Buddha, the twelve hells, and the altars for the souls of the dead had all manifested miraculously!

The monastic brothers and sisters from Prajna had arrived at Soc Son almost a week before the Great Requiem Ceremony began. They had cleaned up the whole area, decorated for the ceremony, and made preparations to cook for the Chanting Masters and all the monastics. Diligent as bees, they were everywhere and working from early morning to late evening.

Prajna brothers and sisters had learned from seeing and helping prepare the decorations for the ceremony at Vinh Nghiem Temple in Saigon, and they used that knowledge to prepare the decorations for this one. Of course, their experience was minimal, and they lacked most of the necessary materials, but because we were taught to "know that you have enough," we could all smile contently. We actually even felt proud!

At first, when I heard the chanting monks stretching out each word at length with "ahh, ahh," I felt anxious. I was afraid that the dead spirits would miss out on the sutras, because fewer actual words were being chanted, and I was afraid that I wouldn't be able to concentrate my mind enough to kneel long hours as I had at Vinh Nghiem and Dieu De. Then I understood that I needed to trust and support these Chanting Masters completely. I opened my heart. Thus, I experienced very joyful and meaningful days there.

All the monastic brothers rested in an abandoned parquet-floored house raised high off the ground. The house had pillars and a roof, but it had no walls, so it was open to the four directions. In the afternoon, the brothers lay down like sardines next to one another to rest from the heat. Someone stretched a hammock between two pillars, enjoying his reading.

The sisters were packed into the two nearby houses. There was no electricity or water. Water had to be pumped and stored in big plastic containers each morning. The two portable toilets were pungent. Yet everyone smiled and spoke joyfully, working together in harmony.

In the early evenings, the brothers went out to play soccer. Only a few hundred meters away from the parquet-floored house, up on the slope, the Buddhist Institute stood, modern and grand.

The night before the Requiem Ceremony began, the Sangha from Prajna invited the monks and nuns from the Buddhist Institute to come down and have a be-in together. Each group explained a few highlights about their practice center.

Brother Trung Hai described three features of Prajna Monastery: "Sixteen people live in the same room. We receive fifty thousand Vietnamese dong (about four US dollars) as our monthly pocket money, and we have no other source of income. We don't have a personal computer or mobile phone."

The groups shared many songs together. The brothers and sisters from the Buddhist Institute expressed their regret that they weren't allowed to house the monastics from Prajna, even though they had plenty of space. However, they sincerely welcomed the Prajna monastics to come up to their quarters, to wash and rest any time during the day. Brotherhood and sisterhood blossomed, and it continued to be nourished in the coming days.

I also stayed at Temple Non with the Prajna sisters, because going back to Bodhi Temple in the city each night would take over an hour and it was too taxing for my health. As long as I had enough space to put down my yoga mat, I was content.

What I minded most at Temple Non was not the eating and sleeping facilities, but the lack of the toilets. There were over ten thousand people attending the Great Requiem Ceremony each day, and we only had a line of portable toilets in the parking lot across the Buddhist Institute. Walking from the area by the parquet-floored house to the parking lot took around fifteen minutes, and from the parking lot to Temple Non took over fifteen minutes, including a steep slope. Given the situation, I decided to minimize eating and drinking, so I wouldn't have to use the toilet as often. However, as it turned out, because I had to go up and down the mountain road three or four times every day, my internal organs were well stimulated, and I ended up needing to use the toilet even more often!

Consequently, one of my missions during those days of the ceremony was to keep a close watch on the two rooms of the monks and the Venerables in the parquet-floored house, because there were toilets inside those rooms. As soon as I saw them empty, I would quickly sneak in to use the toilet. Not only did I do that, but so did all of my sisters and younger brothers. The local Vietnamese laypeople were carefree about relieving themselves in nature along both sides of the road, but our monastics couldn't do that. In talking about our trip to Vietnam, we include our bathroom experience, because it was truly one of the major challenges for us. One time, when some of us were sitting around sharing about memorable events, Brother Phap Son generously praised the bathroom in a Theravadin temple in South Vietnam, which he had visited a few years before. He exclaimed, "That bathroom was so clean, we could have our formal lunch in it!"

Because many people had come from far distant places in the northern region, they had to stay in Temple Non during the three days of the Great Requiem Ceremony. Each night, the elderly and the younger men and women spread out their mats or plastic sheets on the ground, and then lay down closely next to one another. They filled up the veranda and spilled out into the courtyard where there was no roof above them. Children were squeezed in between the adults. People also put chairs together and slept on them. Sister Jina and I looked at the people and smiled. One old woman said, "The monks and nuns are smiling at us!"

Each morning after sitting meditation, Thay took the Sangha on a walking meditation. About a thousand people would be present, but it was completely silent. If there were some newcomers not paying attention and talking, someone in the group would gesture to them to be silent.

On these walks, Thay would turn into the Buddhist Institute, and everyone would follow. The first time this happened, the monks and nuns from the Buddhist Institute stared at us and took many pictures. However, on the last day of the ceremony, they joined us in sitting and walking.

On the way back to Temple Non, Thay stood on the high slope, turned around and looked at the Sangha. Everyone was looking up at him. Thay walked a little further. Then he stopped and looked at the Sangha again. He raised his arms up high, with both hands waving like blooming lotus flowers. Everyone else did the same. I turned to look at the people behind me. Hundreds of bright eyes and joyful smiles, and thousands of hands bloomed like flowers in midair. Thay had often said that children's hands were like flowers. It was in that very moment that I truly touched the beauty of the flower hands. Those hands had held guns and thrown grenades. Those hands had delivered weapons and food on bicycles— everything for the frontline. Now those hands bloomed like flowers, fresh and pure. Someone exclaimed, "If there is healing, healing is taking place right now!"

STUPA OF BROTHERHOOD

On each day of the Great Requiem Ceremony at Temple Non, Thay gave a Dharma talk in the morning with the topic, "My loved ones have died. Where can I find them now?"

It was the same topic as at Temple Vinh Nghiem and Temple Dieu De, but at Temple Non, Thay talked a lot about American soldiers who had survived the Vietnam War. They survived to return to their country, but they were forever haunted by their experiences in Vietnam. Plum Village Monastery had once organized a retreat for Vietnam veterans.

There was a veteran who shared that after all the other soldiers in his troop had been killed, he put gunpowder into sandwiches in order to avenge the soldiers. He placed the sandwiches at the gate of the village and hid himself and watched the village children discovering the sandwiches and eating them. Then the children writhed in agony, and he knew they couldn't be saved, because the hospital was too far away for them to reach it in time. From then on, he couldn't bear to be in the same room with children, even if they were American children.

Another Vietnam veteran shared that he felt afraid when he saw the Sangha doing walking meditation so slowly. It made him remember the days of walking very slowly in tropical jungles to avoid stepping on grenades.

One veteran always carried with him a nylon hammock that belonged to a female guerrilla; she was wounded, and she died in front of him. More than twenty years had passed, but the hatred in her eyes continued to haunt him.

I myself had also worked in Veterans Administration hospitals and had met a number of Vietnam veterans. Most of those young soldiers never recuperated from the war. Many became alcohol and drug dependent. Many were homeless. They developed mental illnesses such as depression, PTSD (post-traumatic stress disorder), and schizophrenia. Now in their fifties, they were overweight, with high blood pressure, diabetes, and other diseases. The northern Vietnamese listened attentively to Thay's stories about Vietnam veterans. Perhaps, they suddenly realized that those veterans, like them, had also been suffering. Perhaps, in a moment of deep understanding and empathy, their hearts opened, and the blocks of hatred and injustices inside them faltered and broke apart.

At the end of his Dharma talk, Thay went directly into the Transmission Ceremony. He read, "This is the moment we transmit the Three Refuges and the Five Mindfulness Trainings. The souls of the dead, please stand up, join your palms, and direct yourselves toward our root teacher, the Buddha." The atmosphere was solemn and silent. Suddenly, there were sounds of chairs pushing and of people standing up. I felt a rush of cold air through my spine. Who had stood up? The living . . . or the dead? Could the souls of the dead ever be removed from the living?

After his final Dharma talk, Thay offered gifts to the Chanting Master and the co-chanters. Instead of giving a single calligraphy to the group, Thay presented a calligraphy to each one of them personally. Thay also offered a calligraphy to the abbot of Temple Non, even though he hadn't been present for the entire ceremony. The Abbot's disciple represented him to receive the calligraphy, and was also given one as well. Thay said to everyone who was present, "I see that a stupa has been erected—a stupa of brotherhood and sisterhood. And this is the highest value of the Great Requiem Ceremony."

The Chan Te ceremony that evening seemed to receive additional energy. The Chanting Master ascended the lion throne, which was directly across from the altar of Amitabha Buddha. The co-chanters sat on both sides of the lion throne. The monastics sat on one side, and laypeople sat all around.

When the dancing monks made the five kinds of offerings to Amitabha Buddha—candlelight, incense, flowers, tea, and fruit—Sister Hanh

Nghiem was the one who received the offerings, one by one, directly from the Chanting Master, and then gave them to the dancing monks. I watched with great interest as Sister Hanh Nghiem assisted the entire ceremony with such aptitude and concentration. She was a pro!

When the chanters prayed for the ten kinds of hungry ghosts, one monk chanted in Sino-Vietnamese, and another monk chanted in Vietnamese, which allowed me to understand the meaning of the words. I translated the chants to the Western brothers and sisters sitting near me, so they could also follow the ceremony. Besides the ten known kinds of hungry ghosts, the monks also chanted about those who did harmful deeds to others, and about those who were attached to their possessions, or to their loved ones, or to other things. The monks began each phrase with, "Then there are the kind of people who . . . " and ended with, "Hungry ghost, oh, dear hungry ghost." Their voices were melancholic and soulful. Suddenly, I gained an insight—that it is our attachments, hatreds, and closed views that imprison us as hungry ghosts, preventing us from going forward and living in the happiness that is available.

Abruptly, the eldest co-chanter made an announcement that caused the chanting to stop midway. He said, "Please remain in order. We still have almost two more hours before the ceremony ends. Even though the Great Requiem Ceremony lasts only three days, it has been in preparation for more than one year, since the Zen Master wrote to ask permission for organizing this ceremony and we were assigned to prepare for it. This Great Ceremony is very rare. These monastics are of the Zen tradition, so please, I ask you to remain peaceful, not causing a ruckus."

The Plum Village monastics smiled at this announcement, because we had learned from the two previous ceremonies that the people in attendance expected to snatch all the food offered to the souls of the dead at the end of the ceremony.

The chanting resumed. The eldest co-chanter interrupted again to ask the people to remain calm. The chanting resumed again, until it was about to end. Brother Phap An began to thank the Chanting Masters; suddenly, there was a loud noise, and the fruit arrangement on the Buddha altar fell down. People shoved each other and snatched whatever they could, on the altar, and on the food tables. It was like a chaotic mob! Brother Phap An spoke up in a louder voice, "As our Teacher has shared, a stupa of brotherhood has been constructed these past few days." He suggested that we sing the song, "I Have Arrived. I Am Home," twice, in English and again in Vietnamese.

All the monastics moved closer to each other and formed a circle. The laypeople continued to push tables and chairs, while the monastics were singing as if nothing else was going on: "I have arrived, I am home, in the here and in the now. I am solid. I am free. In the ultimate, I dwell."

The eldest co-chanter said, "My voice is hoarse from chanting the last three days, but I also want to offer the Plum Village brothers and sisters a song. This is a song we offer to distinguished guests when they come to visit our village."

He began to sing, and all the co-chanters joined him while clapping their hands. The laypeople standing nearby were befuddled by seeing the monastics being so happy together in this situation. They calmed down.

Probably the Chanting Master—who was still sitting on the lion throne—felt that there should be some kind of action, so he began to throw paper money over our heads. He smiled with mischief.

Paper money was falling like leaves, but the laypeople were still and docile! The monastics had to pick up the money and give it to them. Most of the people had already left.

The Chanting Master, the co-chanters, and all the Plum Village and Prajna monastics did walking meditation in a procession back to the building. The area between the Buddha Hall and the building was completely deserted. Some white light from the street was interspersed with the dark night, creating an eerie ambiance. Thousands of people had crowded the place, but now all of them suddenly vanished. There wasn't even one shadow around. I shuddered. Inside the guest room, the monastic brothers were talking and taking pictures joyfully.

FESTIVAL OF A THOUSAND STARS

After our trip was over, Brother Phap Luu shared that one happiness for him after returning to Deer Park Monastery was that, in the morning when he woke up, he could sit still, and he didn't have to take his alms bowl to the bus to go somewhere.

Sister Hanh Nghiem said, "Everyone thinks I'm normal. I eat. I sleep. I use the bathroom. Everything looks normal, but there's something different inside. We experienced something very intense in Vietnam. How can you ever explain that to people?"

I nodded my head in empathy. It has been almost two weeks since I returned to Deer Park, but I continue to limit my contact with people. Even though I have left Vietnam, my mind still has not arrived at Deer Park completely. It is still in a process of digesting and absorbing what I experienced on the journey. I have been using a lot of time to write. I am grateful to the Buddha and to Thay for allowing me to be a monastic. I am grateful that I always have the opportunity to come back to what is happening in the depths of my consciousness, so I may breathe easier, and others may breathe easier.

Spanning a bridge from the cave of hell
all the way to heaven to have a festival of a thousand stars.

ACKNOWLEDGMENTS

The first book that I wrote, *Healing*, was not planned as such. I just wrote journals, letters to Thay, and articles. Then Parallax Press asked me to create a book from these writings.

I never thought of *Healing* as my own. I felt a sense of equanimity about it, that it belongs to the Sangha, not to me, and that it is not about me. If it were about me, I would be embarrassed because it talked about my life. When you talk about your suffering, struggles, challenges, and personal details it can be embarrassing. I felt the book belonged to the Sangha and to the many women and men in the world who have gone through similar experiences.

Healing literally does belong to the Sangha, and all profits go to the Sangha. I have used money from my fifty dollars' monthly allowance to buy copies of the book for close friends and beloved teenagers. When *Healing* first came out in November 2010, we were in Hong Kong with Thay on the Southeast Asia Teaching Tour. Sister Chau Nghiem and I went to the bookstore at our retreat to see the book for the first time. I had borrowed money from one of my monastic brothers to buy the first two copies to offer to Thay and Sister Chan Khong. When the cashier told us the price, I realized that I had borrowed only enough to buy one-and-a-third books. I insisted that they give me a discount. Sister Chau Nghiem pointed to the photo on the back cover and then to my face and said to the cashier, "She wrote this book." Then they agreed to give me a discount. When Thay heard this story, he smiled and said, "This is legendary—the author has to buy her own book!"

I never thought to write a second book. I thought that *Healing* was "it," my contribution to the world, albeit small, but "it contained my intestines, liver, and lungs," as a Vietnamese proverb goes.

However, after I moved to Magnolia Grove Practice Center in Mississippi, I contracted Neuro-Lyme disease from a tick bite, which affected my health severely, and my life changed again.

Due to the unusual, profound, and at times devastating psychological effects caused by this disease, I relived the traumas, losses, and sexual abuses of my early life all over again, and I had to repeat all of the same recuperative steps described in *Healing*, but this time at deeper levels. I learned to love and care for my chronic illness and suffering. In this process I have been exploring more in depth about the teaching on true love for myself and for others.

During the Winter Retreat of 2011–12, Thay said in his Dharma talks that somebody should write a book about true love. That planted a seed in me but, at first, the idea seemed impossible because one of the neurological effects of the Neuro-Lyme disease was to impair my cognitive functions, including speech, writing, and memory. At times, I couldn't spell even simple words. About one year into my illness, my cognitive functions improved tremendously, and Dr. Horowitz literally exclaimed, "It's a miracle!" three times in one office visit. Something deep inside me wanted to share about this experience. The practices of mindfulness and the Six Elements of True Love have helped me to deal with difficulties, challenges, and suffering, to embrace and transform them. I felt blessed to have gone through my illness, and I felt the inspiration and obligation to share what I had learned with others.

One day, as I was listening to Thay's Dharma talk, the idea came to me that if a new book could not be written by me directly because of my cognitive dysfunction, it might still be voice recorded, transcribed, and edited later. Sister Truc Nghiem devoted her monastic Lazy Days to interviewing me. Uncle Lam Nguyen, Anne Speiser, and Stephanie Davies helped to transcribe the text. Uncle Gene Kira with his "beautiful mind" helped edit and put all of my writings together into the first manuscript with deep care and understanding. Jennifer Ruby Privateer, Terri Saul, and Rachel Neumann generously helped with the final manuscript. Thus, this book is a collective project. It's also a collective insight because it draws from the experiences of many people and from lessons I have learned from myself and from them.

I am grateful to all the people I have met in my life, especially in my monastic life thus far. I share with them the mindfulness practice and my own experience with healing. At the same time, my encounter with them also helps me to see my own mind more clearly and to take better care of myself.

In this book, I would like to acknowledge the stories of all the people who have made a difference in my process of healing. However, there are many stories that I'm not able to recount here. Even if I don't have the opportunity to ask these people for permission to share their stories, I hope that they will accept this book as an offering to the world, to help make the healing of many others possible. The healing of one person can heal many because we inter-are.

As a nun, I don't have much in the material world. The most I have had in my possession sometimes has been a few hundred dollars and a few robes. Yet I am able to look at myself. When I lie down to sleep, I can say to myself that if I don't wake up, it will be okay and I will have no regret. I don't see that I have left the field of medicine. To me, mindfulness is the most profound medicine that I can apply in my daily life, to take care of myself, to transform and heal the suffering in myself, and thus, it's also the greatest medicine that I may offer to others.

This is the work of a bridge-builder that I would like to dedicate my life to, sharing concrete experiences and practices so that others may be able to avoid some perilous paths that I have crossed, to transform their suffering, and to experience true love. I hope this message will be accessible to teenagers as well as people of all ages, regardless of religious and cultural backgrounds.

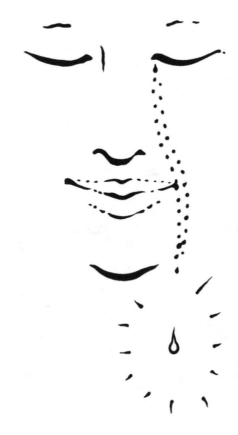

a drop of tear
and a gentle smile
born
at the same instant
and a heart is forever changed

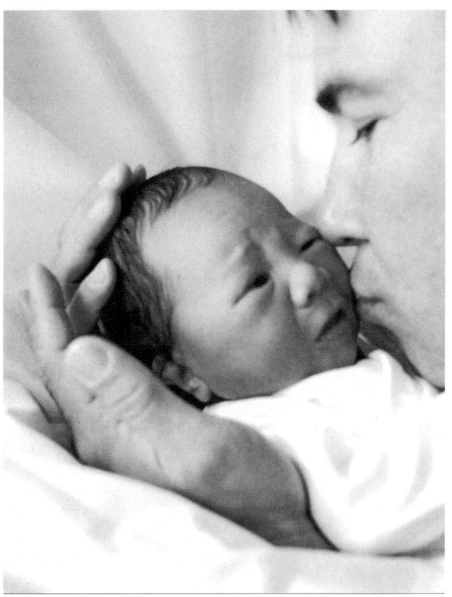

BROTHER SONNY & HIS DAUGHTER SUNEE

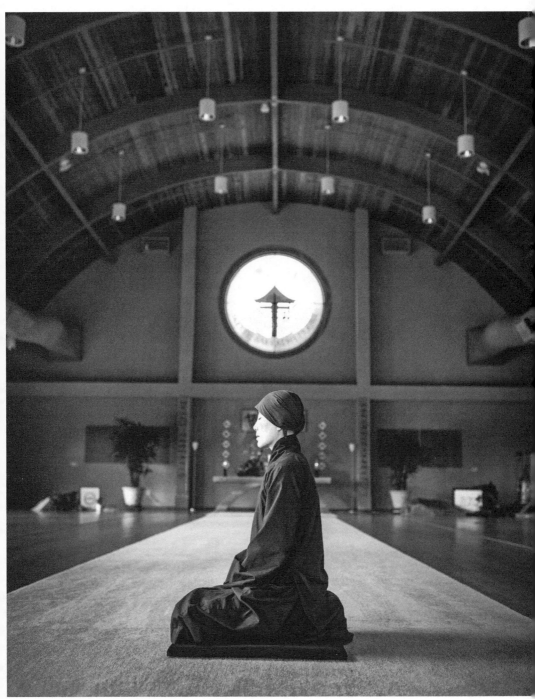

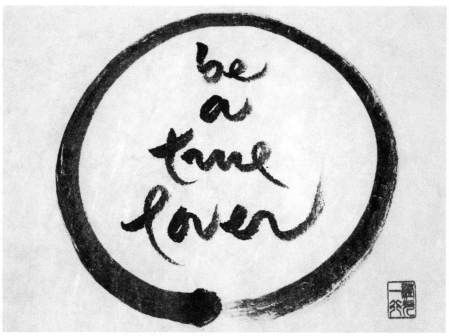

RELATED TITLES

A Mindful Way Jeannie Seward-Magee

Beginning Anew Sister Chan Khong

Cultivating the Mind of Love Thich Nhat Hanh

The Energy of Prayer Thich Nhat Hanh

First Buddhist Women Susan Murcott

Healing Sister Dang Nghiem

Learning True Love Sister Chan Khong

Not Quite Nirvana Rachel Neumann

Pass It On Joanna Macy

Reconciliation Thich Nhat Hanh

Teachings on Love Thich Nhat Hanh

Ten Breaths to Happiness Glen Schneider

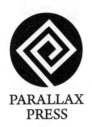

PARALLAX
PRESS

Parallax Press is a nonprofit publisher, founded and inspired by Zen Master Thich Nhat Hanh. We publish books on mindfulness in daily life and are committed to making these teachings accessible to everyone and preserving them for future generations. We do this work to alleviate suffering and contribute to a more just and joyful world.

For a copy of the catalog, please contact:

Parallax Press
P.O. Box 7355
Berkeley, CA 94707
Tel: (510) 525-0101
parallax.org

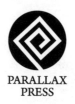

PARALLAX
PRESS

Parallax Press, a nonprofit organization, publishes books on engaged Buddhism and the practice of mindfulness by Thich Nhat Hanh and other authors. All of Thich Nhat Hanh's work is available at our online store and in our free catalog. For a copy of the catalog, please contact:

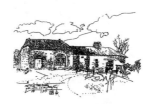

Parallax Press
P.O. Box 7355
Berkeley, CA 94707
Tel: (510) 525-0101
parallax.org

Monastics and laypeople practice the art of mindful living in the tradition of Thich Nhat Hanh at retreat communities worldwide. To reach any of these communities, or for information about individuals and families joining for a practice period, please contact:

Plum Village
13 Martineau
33580 Dieulivol, France
plumvillage.org

Blue Cliff Monastery
3 Mindfulness Road
Pine Bush, NY 12566
bluecliffmonastery.org

Magnolia Grove Monastery
123 Towles Rd.
Batesville, MS 38606
magnoliagrovemonastery.org

Deer Park Monastery
2499 Melru Lane
Escondido, CA 92026
deerparkmonastery.org

The Mindfulness Bell, a journal of the art of mindful living in the tradition of Thich Nhat Hanh, is published three times a year by Plum Village. To subscribe or to see the worldwide directory of Sanghas, visitmindfulnessbell.org.